Isaac Ray

Mental Hygiene

Isaac Ray

Mental Hygiene

ISBN/EAN: 9783741123306

Manufactured in Europe, USA, Canada, Australia, Japa

Cover: Foto ©Lupo / pixelio.de

Manufactured and distributed by brebook publishing software
(www.brebook.com)

Isaac Ray

Mental Hygiene

MENTAL HYGIENE

BY

I. RAY, M. D.,

Health of mind, as well as of body, is not only productive in itself of a greater sum of enjoyment than arises from other sources, but is the only condition of our frame in which we are capable of receiving pleasure from without. — SIR JAMES MACKINTOSH.

BOSTON:
TICKNOR AND FIELDS.
1863.

ADVERTISEMENT.

THE present work is not offered as a systematic treatise on Mental Hygiene. Its purpose is mainly to expose the mischievous effects of many practices and customs prevalent in modern society, and to present some practical suggestions relative to the attainment of mental soundness and vigor. If it shall lead, in any degree, to serious reflection and amendment, its object will have been well accomplished.

*a**

CONTENTS.

———

CHAPTER I.

MENTAL HYGIENE AS AFFECTED BY CEREBRAL CONDITIONS.

CHAPTER II.

MENTAL HYGIENE AS AFFECTED BY PHYSICAL IN-
FLUENCES.

CHAPTER III.

MENTAL HYGIENE AS AFFECTED BY MENTAL CONDITIONS AND INFLUENCES.

CHAPTER IV.

MENTAL HYGIENE AS AFFECTED BY THE PRACTICES OF THE TIMES.

CHAPTER V.

MENTAL HYGIENE AS AFFECTED BY TENDENCY TO DISEASE.

MENTAL HYGIENE.

CHAPTER. I.

MENTAL HYGIENE AS AFFECTED BY CEREBRAL CON-
DITIONS.

FEW, even of those who are accustomed to
think and inquire, recognize, fully and practically, the important truth that the efficiency of
the mental powers is determined in a high degree by the hygienic condition of the bodily
organs, especially the brain. This organ has always been regarded as somehow necessary to
the mental manifestations, but beyond this single
fact, there has been noticed scarcely any other
indication of their mutual dependence. Indeed,
the spiritual element of the mind has seemed to
place it beyond the accidents of health and disease. Besides, the idea that it could be affected
by any merely physical conditions seemed to be
degrading to its dignity, and indicative of the
coarsest materialism. If the mind may be diseased, then it may perish, and so our hopes of

1

immortality be utterly destroyed. This startling
conclusion has been sufficient to deter the mass
of mankind from admitting very heartily the
facts which physiological and pathological inquiries have contributed to this subject. The
people who have no difficulty in discerning the
relation between the health of the lungs and the
atmospherical conditions around them, or between the health of the digestive organs and the
food they are expected to elaborate, utterly ignore all connection between the hygienic condition of the brain and the mental energies dependent upon it. Thus they completely missed the
principle which is the foundation of all true mental hygiene, viz. that the manifestations of the
mind and the organic condition of the brain are
more or less affected by each other.

The conditions of this relation, — the parts respectively borne by the bodily and the spiritual
element in the production of the mental manifestations, — of course, are but imperfectly understood. And perhaps much of the reluctance to
accept and apply the facts which physiological
and pathological inquiries have contributed to
this subject, may be traced to a fear of the materialism which they were too readily supposed
to imply. The difficulty always has been so to
define the limits between the physical and the
spiritual, as to secure to man the exclusive pos-

session of a high prerogative. If the mind is the only part destined to be immortal, it seemed to be necessary, in order to avoid an unpleasant conclusion, that it should be so defined as to exclude any manifestations of the brutes. Hence have arisen countless speculations more ingenious than sound concerning the nature of mind; and hence it is, too, that after all that has been said and written, the current philosophy on the subject does not fairly represent the facts of science. What we know as certain is contained within a very small compass, and may be briefly considered before entering upon the task before us, in order, especially, to prevent any misunderstanding as to the meaning of common terms and modes of expression.

The *mind*, as I understand it, embraces all the powers, qualities, and attributes, which are concerned in maintaining those relations to other beings that are necessary to our highest welfare. The faculty which investigates the relations of cause and effect is not more truly a manifestation of mind, than the power to love and to hate. Whether we meditate on lofty truths, or on the beautiful creations of the painter and sculptor; whether we recognize and revere the claims of superior virtue, or burn with desire to revenge a wrong; whether we yield to the allurements of love, or start with horror from impending destruction,— in each and every instance, we manifest some quality of mind. Like the flower, like the insect, like the crystal, like every work of God, the mind is complete and perfect in its kind. Every one of its powers is designed to accomplish some indispensable purpose, and bears the marks of unerring wisdom. Unlike the works just mentioned, however, it is susceptible of indefinite development, whereby it becomes capable of fulfilling the nobler ends of our existence.

In this life, at least, the mental powers are connected, in some way, with the brain. On this point all are agreed, but, as to the nature of this connection, there has always been the greatest possible variety of opinion. The most prevalent belief, both among the wise and the simple, is that the mind is an independent essence or principle requiring the brain, not for its existence, but only for the mode of its manifestation. As the music is in the player, not in the instrument he uses, so is the brain the material organ by which the mind is enabled to exercise its powers. On the other hand, among men whose views on philosophical subjects are determined more by the testimony of sense than any subtle deductions of reason, there are some who regard the mind as entirely a function of the brain. Without the brain there is, and there can be, no mind. This question, as already hinted, derives

its importance chiefly from its theological bearings. If the mind is an original, independent
principle having only an incidental connection
with the body, then, it is supposed, it may, and
indeed must exist after the dissolution of the
body. But, if it is merely a phenomenon resulting from the play of organic elements, it must
necessarily perish with the organism from which
it sprung. It is not quite certain that either
of these views will warrant the inference that is
drawn from it. Although we may admit the independent existence of the mind, there must be
other reasons, I apprehend, for believing it to be
immortal; and, though we may admit that the
mind is a product of vital movements, it does not
necessarily follow that there can be no conscious
existence after the component parts of the animal mechanism are dispersed. We are not to
measure the resources of Almighty Power by our
own feeble conceptions, nor to suppose that a
fact is impossible merely because some of its
conditions are beyond our comprehension.

In this question is involved another of a more
practical character, viz. is the *development* of
the mind a result exclusively spiritual, or exclusively cerebral? When a person has grown
wiser and better with ripening age, has the
change been effected by increasing the delicacy
of the organism, or by developing the faculties

independently of any such process? When the
mental traits of the offspring resemble the parent's, is it the physical or the spiritual element,
that has been transmitted? We know too little
of the connection between mind and body to answer these questions very definitely. Each sup-
position is burdened with difficulties that indicate some radical defect in the common philosophy on this subject. It may be doubted if it is
quite correct to consider the individual as composed of two things essentially distinct both in
origin and nature, instead of regarding him as
a being endowed with various powers which,
though serving each a special purpose, form an
harmonious whole — a single, individual man.

The difficulty of explaining upon the common theory the facts that meet us at every turn,
little as it may seem in some instances, is perfectly insuperable in others. When a sinner is
suddenly turned from his wicked courses by an
awakening appeal, or a painter has embodied
upon the canvas some new-born conception of
his fancy, it is obviously a practical absurdity
to suppose that these persons have only experienced some change in the arrangement of the
organic particles of the brain. Equally absurd
would it seem, to suppose that the disease, or
injury, or old age, which has impaired the vigor
of the intellect, acted immediately on the men-

tal powers, leaving the nervous system endowed
with all its original integrity and delicacy. In
the cases here indicated, there can be no difference of opinion; but who would venture to
make the requisite distinction in all the countless movements that constitute the mental life
of the individual, ranging from the transitory
emotions of the child to the profoundest deductions of the philosopher? And in those cases
where we think we witness both a corporeal
and a spiritual movement, who shall undertake
to assign the part respectively borne by each?
When a choleric mortal becomes red in the face,
and foams with rage under the sense of insult
or injury; or a troop of jolly companions are
making merry over their liquor, we are accustomed to say that a movement of blood to the
brain or a fresh impulse of the nervous current,
has given rise to a strong mental emotion, but
beyond the simplest statement of the fact we
can say nothing, though quite sure that this is
not the only agency in the case. On the other
hand, when we see the accomplished orator
swaying at his will the convictions and passions
of a vast assembly, we call it a triumph of mind;
but we are obliged to admit that it is accompanied by an unwonted degree of cerebral activity. This doctrine of the unity of the individual man, as applied to the subject of mental

hygiene, obliges us to be content with the general principle, that whatever improves the physical qualities of the brain also improves, in some
way or other, the qualities of the mind; and that
judicious exercise of the mind is followed by
the same result. In both cases, in fact, we observe the same law of development whereby the
systematic and appropriate exercise of a part is
followed by increased vigor, capacity, and power
of endurance, while a deficient or excessive exercise is followed by weakness and premature
decay.

Another point touching the connection of
mind and body demands a passing notice in
these preliminary remarks. The simple fact that
the brain is the material instrument of the mind
has not always satisfied those who were familiar
with its structure. When they looked on the
intricate convolutions of its surface, and observed its division into hemispheres and lobes;
when with knife in hand they exposed its various rounded masses of nervous matter, and
traced the medullary bands that united one side
with the other; when they unfolded its ventri-
cles and followed the sensorial nerves to their
origin, they could scarcely help conceiving the
idea that the different parts of the wonderful
organ before them must have each its particular
office in the work of manifesting the mind. It

was reserved for our own day, however, to see this speculation assume the shape of a complete and systematic body of doctrine, in which every portion of the cortical substance of the brain is assigned to some particular faculty, sentiment, or propensity, each of which is regarded as an original, innate, independent power, exercised by its appropriate organ. In the localization of these organs the founders of Phrenology profess to have been guided solely by observation; but they also endeavor, in every instance, to show that the necessities of the human economy require such a power. In the latter branch of their system, they have been more fortunate, perhaps, than in the former. In a few instances, both the existence and the place of the organ have been established by abundant proof; but, with these exceptions, the evidence has not satisfied the deliberate and unbiassed judgment of scientific men. As a speculative theory, it unquestionably contains much truth, recognized as such, too, by many who have little sympathy with its anatomical doctrines. Its analysis of the mental phenomena is clear and precise, indicating — what metaphysical inquiries seldom have — a shrewd observation of the springs of action, and a profound insight of the relations of man to the sphere in which he moves. Deficient as it is, as a theory of mind, it is neverthe-

less valuable as having indicated the true mode
of investigation, and especially for the light it
throws on the whole process of education and
development.

It is proper, in this connection, to consider
that the essential ends and objects of our existence are not left to the accidents of education,
but are provided for in the very constitution of
our nature. Such a provision, whether in the
shape of an animal propensity, an all-prevailing
sentiment or belief, or a special aptitude and
ability, must be regarded as conclusive proof of
the reality and importance of the end thus secured. Every sentiment or power must have its
means of gratification, or field of exercise. To
suppose the contrary would be as repugnant to
every idea of moral fitness as that fancy of the
poets which attributed sensation to the trees,
though without the power of pursuing pleasure
or avoiding pain. That sentiment which impels
us to shrink from death, and cling to life however burdened with sorrow, we call an original
sentiment of our nature, required for that indispensable end, the preservation of the individual.
With equal reason we may say that the longing
for existence beyond the present life — the conviction, not derived from philosophy or poetry,
that this is not the be-all and the end-all with
us — is an original sentiment of our nature, and

thus proves the reality of the existence which its gratification requires. We must adopt this conclusion, or believe that the mind, so perfect in every other respect, is at fault here — endowed with a power which has no possible sphere of activity. It may be said that this is one of those' convictions which result from education, and consequently has none of that certainty which belongs to an original sentiment. The premise may be partly true, and the conclusion false. We admit the fact that the sentiment in question, not being necessary to the preservation of the individual, sometimes gives but faint tokens of its presence, because development is required to make it a quickening principle, inspiring him with loftier aims and pointing to a nobler destiny than any which the largest experience of life could reveal. The nerves are not originally endowed with that delicacy of feeling, nor the muscles with that degree of power which training is capable of conferring; but it is no less true that these organs are possessed by the infant as well as the full-grown man.

The limits within which mental cultivation may produce its appropriate effects have not always been very correctly defined. Some of the elements of the question are beyond our reach; but, in regard to others, our knowledge is abundant, and there can scarcely be any diversity of

opinion. Cultivation of the bodily and mental
powers raises the individual to a higher point
in the scale of being ; and, of course, the more
widely it is diffused the greater will be the number of those who achieve this elevation. The
effect in question is not merely an increase of
knowledge with its accompanying benefits, but
an enlargement of all those qualities on which
the efficiency of the mind depends. It is exemplified in the difference between a native Aus-
tralian and a cultivated European ; between
the unthinking multitude and the Bacons and
Newtons of the world. Individuals of the former classes may be improved, but no ingenuity
of discipline could possibly raise them to the
level of the latter. The only question is whether
any point of development reached by the individual may be regarded as a step established
and secured towards the indefinite elevation of
the race ; whether, in other words, the improvement of the individual may not become congenital in his offspring, and thus furnish a new
starting-point, at every remove, for higher advancement. In reply, we need only refer to the
well recognized laws which govern the transmission of qualities in the inferior animals. These
laws warrant the belief that, by complying with
their requirements, the traits of the individual,
mental as well as bodily, may be made perma-

nent in the race, with such limitations as are imposed by the distinctive character of the species. Under any possible improvement of this kind, man must still remain a man — he cannot become a demigod or an angel.

We must distinctly understand what can and what cannot be accomplished by a faithful compliance with the laws of breeding. We are entirely destitute of any experiments on the subject, but we have no reason to believe from analogy that the mind can be lifted to higher grades of excellence than it has already reached. The remarkable quality which stock-breeders succeed in rendering permanent in the domestic animals — fleetness in one, power in another, size in another, a certain relation between bone and muscle in another — represents but a small fraction of the whole constitution. The fleet Arabian cannot be considered as nearer the point of equine perfection than the immense English dray-horse; nor would any one but a Smithfield drover contend that a Berkshire or a Suffolk is a worthier specimen of the porcine race than the wild boar of the forest. Thus the question as to the extent to which improvement of the race may be carried cannot be settled by these results in the arts of breeding, which indicate only partial elevation. There has not yet been obtained in any particular breed a considerable number

of desirable qualities; for the general rule is
that each special excellence is obtained at the
expense of some other. So well is this now understood, that nobody attempts to obtain in one
breed the excellences of all. Now, what we seek
for as the proper result and aim of mental cultivation is, not a particular endowment that may
be transmitted from one generation to another,
but a large range of capacity, great facility of
achievement, and great power of endurance.
That these qualities may be rendered permanent by a faithful compliance with the laws of
breeding, there can scarcely be a doubt; but
this, it must be observed, is something very far
short of indefinite development. We have no
reason to suppose that, by any possible scheme
of training and breeding, finer specimens of the
race can be obtained than Pericles and Alcibia-
des; but we are warranted in believing that by
this means individuals of distinguished general
excellence would be far more common. If it be
true, then, that, in the various stages of its progress, the mind, like the body, is under the government of inflexible laws, it follows that these
laws should be thoroughly understood, in order
to obtain the highest possible degree of mental
efficiency. To show exactly what they are, to
exhibit the consequences that flow from obeying
or disobeying them, is the essential object of

MENTAL HYGIENE, which may be defined as the
art of preserving the health of the mind against
all the incidents and influences calculated to
deteriorate its qualities, impair its energies, or
derange its movements. The management of
the bodily powers in regard to exercise, rest,
food, clothing, and climate ; the laws of breeding,
the government of the passions, the sympathy
with current emotions and opinions, the discipline of the intellect, — all come within the province of mental hygiene. A complete and scientific treatise on the subject would require
discussions, details, and references, of little interest to the general reader, for whom this work is
chiefly designed. I shall aim to present only
the general conclusions that have been reached,
with no more of detail than is necessary to make
the matter intelligible and impress it the more
strongly on the mind.

In using the term, *mind*, in the following
pages, I shall not restrict myself to its popular
meaning, as something separate and distinct
from the body, but shall employ it as a generic
expression of the mental phenomena without
reference to their origin or nature. And so of
the term, *brain*. However I may use it for the
sake of convenience, I would not be supposed
to favor any theory whatever respecting its connection with the mind. Being the instrument

of the mind, its condition must necessarily affect the mental manifestations, and therefore it may not be improper to speak of mental disorders as if the brain were the only agency concerned in them.

Now, more than ever before, the fortunes of men, the welfare and happiness of the race, are determined by mental efficiency. The time has been when the mass of the people had but little use for their minds. They had no occasion to think. Indeed they were forbidden to think. A few favored mortals did their thinking for them. It was enough for them to do as they were bid. Stout limbs, stalwart frames, robust health, were what the times demanded and what the times admired. A man was valued by the force of his blows, by his swiftness of foot, by his capacity for hardship. Now, these qualities will give him but a low place in the social scale, and secure for him but a small share of those privileges which constitute the highest kind of human happiness. Never before did so large a portion of mankind think. Never before did so large a portion of the race strive together for the great prizes of life, in a contest of mind with mind, not muscle with muscle, nor limb with limb — a contest in which, in the long run, the mind will win that can accomplish the greatest amount of work. I use the phrase advisedly.

We are so much in the habit of believing that great intellects alone are capable of great achievements, that we get the idea that minds less happily endowed can make no impression on the world. Leaving out of view the splendid exceptional cases, the careful observer can hardly avoid the conclusion, that the original endowment has less to do with the result, than the patient application, the indomitable perseverance, the unwearied endurance. Great geniuses come by nature. What we want — what, I believe, is within the reach of the race — are healthy, vigorous, well-balanced minds. Let us then consider some of the principal incidents and conditions on which these qualities depend ; and first, those of an outward or physical character.

There are two indispensable requisites to a sound and vigorous mind, viz. a brain free from all congenital tendencies to disease or deterioration, and a healthy condition of the other bodily organs. The first results from a rigid compliance with the laws of breeding, which regulate the transmission of organic traits and qualities from one generation to another. Men are too apt to imagine that these laws have no other end than that of preserving the characters of the species, entirely overlooking that other indispensable end, the preservation of the characters of the individual. The

2

truth is that not only are the forms of the body thus maintained within certain rigorous limits of variation, but also its hygienic conditions, for good or for ill. If the progenitors have been sound and vigorous, other things being equal, so will be the offspring. If the former have been afflicted with disease or physical imperfection, so will be many of the latter.

One of the most prolific sources of mental unsoundness or imperfection, is the existence of insanity or remarkable eccentricity, in some previous generation. No fact in nature is better established than this, — that a large proportion of the offspring of persons who have been insane or highly eccentric at some time or other, become insane or eccentric to a degree little short of insanity. In every hospital for the insane, it will be found that at least one half the patients are of this description; and there can be no doubt, if the history of the other half were better known, that this proportion would be greatly raised. Seldom does it happen that this infirmity of the fathers fails altogether to be visited upon the children. It may skip over a whole generation, and make its appearance in the next. It may be gross eccentricity in the parent, and overt, unmistakable derangement in the descendant; and *vice versa.* The predisposition may be transmitted irrespective of other parental qualities; and the child who bears the features exclusively of the father may inherit the mother's tendency to disease. It may strike down its victim in the freshness and vigor of youth ; it may wait until the mind has stood many a shock and passed through many a trial.

To those who are yet to form the most important of all connections in life, the facts here stated speak in tones of solemn admonition, warning them, by all their hopes of domestic happiness, against disregarding a law which carries with it such fearful penalties. The highest mental and personal accomplishments will prove to be no compensation for the evil ; nor will they furnish any excuse for compromising the welfare of those who derive from us their existence. None but they who have a professional acquaintance with the subject can conceive of the amount of wretchedness in the world produced by this single cause. None can adequately estimate the suffering, the privation, the ruined hopes, the crushed affections, the blighted prospects, that may be fairly numbered among its effects.

The mental constitution may be vitiated by the presence in the progenitors of other diseases than insanity, especially epilepsy, hysteria, chorea, scrofula, rickets. This effect may not appear in the shape of positive disease, though that

is not uncommon. It may often be witnessed
in a reduction of the moral and intellectual capacity, and a remarkable activity and prominence
of the animal propensities. In persons thus
affected, the voice of conscience is feeble, the
restraints of law are powerless, vice is far more
congenial than virtue, and temptation always
obtains an easy conquest. The same traits of
character are not unfrequently witnessed by the
careful observer of men, in those classes of people who, for several generations, have been exposed to those physical agencies which, by
depressing the vital energies and preventing the
full, rounded development of the system, deteriorate the qualities of the brain. The history of
the individual will show that these traits are not
the results of casual circumstances, nor of special
training, but are of spontaneous growth, and
but little affected by those benignant influences
that never fail to improve the character, in some
degree, in persons of a healthier organization.
The effect in question has been observed on a
large scale, in some of the old cities of Europe,
where the causes are peculiarly active and
abundant. The bad air, the excessive cold
and heat and moisture which characterize the
localities of the poor, and the lack of nutritious
food, especially in childhood, not only give rise
to fever and other epidemics, but vitiate the very

springs of life, and produce debility, distortion, and unbalanced activity, to be transmitted in greater intensity to the offspring. A healthy, well-balanced brain, under such circumstances, must be the exception, not the rule. As well might we look among the growth of a thickly-planted grove for the full development and fine proportions of the noble tree standing out alone upon the lawn, exposed to the air and light of heaven, and nourished by a fertile soil.

These results are still more obvious where the low grade of moral and physical endow-ment thus produced is accompanied by a ten-dency to insanity, derived from progenitors. Under such circumstances, the mental deterio-ration is characterized by a strong proclivity to vice and crime, that cannot be explained by any circumstances of education. A complete his-tory of the inmates of our jails and prisons, embracing all their antecedents, would show, in regard to a large portion of them, that the active element was not immoral training, nor extraor-dinary temptations, but defective cerebral en-dowment traceable to the agencies here men-tioned. They enter upon life with a cerebral organization deficient in those qualities neces-sary for the manifestation of the higher mental functions. Many of them are bad subjects

from the cradle, and their whole life is a series
of aggressions on their fellow-men. Whether
they finish their career in a hospital or a prison, is
a point oftener decided by adventitious circumstances than any definite, well-settled principles.
The frequency of insanity among convicts in
prison is, probably, not so much owing to the
immediate circumstances of their position, as to
this latent element of mischief in their mental
constitution, which, no doubt, is rendered more
active by confinement.

When the physical defects of the parent are
entailed upon the offspring in the shape of de-
formity and disease, they excite no other emotions than those of pity, and a disposition to relieve. Without discussing the question, whether
a person whose heritage of infirmity consists in
a defective brain should be held to a rigid responsibility for the consequences of his misfortune, rather than regarded with the same emotions, I apprehend there can be no diversity of
opinion as to the importance of the facts in
connection with the subject of social morality.
For the moral and intellectual elevation of the
race, we are to look, not exclusively to education, but to whatever tends to improve the
bodily constitution, and especially the qualities
of the brain. In our schemes of philanthropy,

we are apt to deal with men as if they could be moulded to any desirable purpose, provided only the right instrumentalities are used; ignoring altogether the fact, that there is a physical organ in the case, whose original endowments must limit very strictly the range of our moral appliances. But while we are bringing to bear upon them all the kindly influences of learning and religion, let us not overlook those physical agencies which determine the efficiency of the brain as the material instrument of the mind. The tract and the missionary may do good service in the dwellings of the ignorant and depraved, but active ventilation, thorough sewerage, abundance of water, will be found, eventually, no less efficient in the work of reform and elevation. To check the increase of crime, improve, if you please, your penal legislation and penal discipline, but, above all things, improve the dwellings of the poor. Render industry and virtue as attractive as possible, but never cease, by all practicable means, to prevent the production of tubercle, rickets, scrofula, and all defective or unequal developments. Encourage frugality and forecast, but discourage, by every consideration that science has furnished, the marriage of the infirm, the sickly, and the deformed.

The great practical neglect of this organic

law of hereditary transmission, and its recent denial in a work of remarkable ability, induce us to state very briefly what the doctrine really is, and the evidence on which it rests.

The law which pervades the propagation of living beings, preserving the unity of the species, and setting bounds to accidental or abnormal variations, is, that like produces like. Thus, through successive ages, the characters that mark the species are preserved, and the order and harmony of nature maintained. But a certain amount of variety is not inconsistent with harmony, and, therefore, individuals, while agreeing in all the characters of the species, are distinguished from one another by some obvious though subordinate traits of difference. In animate objects, perfect identity is no more a part of Nature's arrangements than unlimited variety. In every individual, therefore, we have two different orders of characters; one which he possesses in common with all other individuals of his species, and another which are peculiar to himself or a few others. That the former are preserved by hereditary transmission, of course, nobody doubts, and the fact shows the possibility, if it does not afford presumptive proof, that the latter are governed by the same law. Such, certainly, is the ordinary belief, as it regards the normal physical traits of family resemblance,

but it is now contended that moral and intellectual qualities, and even diseases or tendencies to disease, are not so transmitted, — that,
when possessed by both parent and offspring,
the coincidence is merely accidental.* This
view of the subject seems to arise from a mis-
conception of some of the conditions which attend the operation of the law. It is alleged that
if it were one of the laws of generation, that
the traits in question are transmitted from parent to offspring, it ought to be a matter of more
common occurrence; whereas, instances of this
kind of resemblance are greatly outnumbered
by those of diversity. The general fact, certainly, is true, though not perhaps to the extent here
implied, but it does not disprove this kind of hereditary transmission. It is no part of the doctrine that such transmission is uniform and universal. If it were, we should have equal reason
to believe that resemblance of physical features,
form, complexion, countenance, is also accidental, because frequently, in these respects, the
child is quite unlike the parent. Considering
the tendency of nature to infinite diversity in
its works, the instances of resemblance that
do occur, though bearing but a small proportion,
perhaps, to those of a different character, force
us to conclude that the coincidence is not acci-

* Buckle, T., *History of Civilization*, I. 161.

dental, but the result of a general law. Constant, invariable coincidence could not be
expected, when we consider that hereditary
transmission is under the control of a double
law, whereby the type of the species as well as
of the family is maintained. Even under the
widest deviations from the normal type, there is
ever a tendency to regain the original characters
of the race. A trait which distinguishes two or
three successive generations may be scarcely
observed in the fourth, and finally be lost altogether. It may appear in one member of the
family, and be absent from another. A trait
which distinguishes one generation may be entirely wanting in the next, and reappear in the
third.

There is another reason, and a very efficient
one, why the peculiarities of the parent should
not be invariably transmitted to the offspring.
The child has a double origin, drawing its family traits from two different sources. The manner in which the two parents are represented in
the offspring is subject to considerable diversity.
The peculiar marks of one of them may greatly
predominate over those of the other, and even
exclude them altogether; or they may mingle
together with some approach to equality. The
parents themselves have inherited the traits of
their progenitors, which may be more fully

evolved in their offspring than in themselves, and thus the child is made to represent many individuals besides the immediate authors of its being. Thus it is, that the complete transmission of the peculiarities of the two parents is simply impossible; and the happy consequence of such extensive intermixture in the product of generation is, that peculiarities — especially those of a morbid or abnormal character — are finally absorbed in the characters that constitute the type of the species.

Against the doctrine of the hereditary character of some diseases, it is objected that the legitimate effect of such an organic law would be to deteriorate the human constitution, until every trace of its original stamina shall have disappeared. Of course, the same disease is often seen in both parent and child, but this is regarded as only a casual concidence. This objection is founded upon a very incorrect idea of the laws of hereditary transmission, as might be inferred from the statement at the close of the last paragraph. The transmission of disease is modified by the same class of agencies as the transmission of feature, or temperament, or complexion. We have no more right to expect that the insanity, or scrofula, or hare-lip of the parent should be transmitted to every one of his children, than we have to expect that a prominent chin, or a large frame, or a dark complexion should be thus transmitted. The tendency, already spoken of, to regain the normal type after the most considerable deviations, is even more obvious in the case of disease and anomalous formation than in that of ordinary peculiarities. Besides, we are to recollect that it is not necessarily the disease which is transmitted, but only the predisposition to disease, and this, owing to some fortunate conjunction of circumstances, may never be developed into overt disease. Two brothers, for instance, may have inherited a tendency to insanity. One is exposed to circumstances that try the mental energies beyond the power of endurance, and he becomes insane. The other pursues the voyage of life on a tranquil sea, with favoring gales, and thus avoids altogether the impending blow. True, instances where the disease of the child has apparently been derived from the parent, may be perhaps outnumbered by those where there has obviously been no such transmission. But this would not help the objection, unless we alleged that the diseases in question had no other origin than that of hereditary transmission. They may be derived from the parent, or from agencies that supervened subsequent to birth. These two different orders of fact are not incompatible, as all the analogies of nature show. To deny the

hereditary character of some diseases, merely
because they are not always hereditary, is no
better philosophy than it would be to believe
that scarlatina, typhus, measles, glanders, are
never contagious because by the side of cases
which seem to have originated in contagion are
many that cannot be traced to this cause.

That the soundness and vigor of the human
constitution are greatly impaired by the hereditary transmission of disease can scarcely be
doubted by those who have been much conversant with the subject, and though any approach
to thorough and universal deterioration has been
avoided by that beneficent law whereby the
normal type of the species prevails sooner or
later, under favorable circumstances, over all
casual deviations, yet the evil is serious and extensive enough, it might be supposed, to induce
the wise and prudent, if no others, to avoid the
causes which produce it.

Let us, however, avoid the common error of
supposing that under the law of hereditary transmission the abnormal trait of the parent, and
that only, is exactly repeated in the offspring.
The only essential element of the hereditary act
is defect, deterioration, or vitiated quality of the
brain. What phasis it may finally assume, depends on conditions beyond the reach of our
knowledge. We might as well expect to see

the eyes or the nose, the figure or the motions of either parent transmitted with the exactest likeness to all the offspring, as to suppose that an hereditary disease must necessarily be transmitted fully formed, with all the incidents and conditions which it possessed in the parent. And yet in the case of mental disease, the current philosophy can recognize the evidence of transmission in no shape less demonstrative than delusion or raving. Contrary to all analogy and contrary to all fact, it supposes that the hereditary affection must appear in the offspring in precisely the same degree of intensity which it had in the parent. If the son is stricken down with raving mania, like his father before him, then the relation of cause and effect is obvious enough; but if, on the contrary, the former exhibits only extraordinary outbreaks of passion, remarkable inequalities of spirit and disposition, irrelevant and inappropriate conduct, strange and unaccountable impulses, nothing of this kind is charged to the parental infirmity. Such views are not warranted by the present state of our knowledge respecting the hereditary transmission of disease.

There is a phasis of hereditary transmission, which it may be well to advert to, because though not very uncommon it is far from being properly understood. The transmitted defect is confined

to a very circumscribed range, beyond which the
mind presents no obvious impairment. The
sound and the unsound coexist, not in a state of
fusion, but side by side, each independent of the
other, and both derived from a common source.
And the fact is no more anomalous than that often witnessed, of some striking feature of one
parent associated in the child with one equally
striking of the other. It is not the case exactly,
of partial insanity, or any mental defect, superin-
duced upon a mind otherwise sound, for such defect is, in some degree, an accident, and may
disappear; but here is a congenital conjunction
of sanity and insanity, which no medical or
moral appliances will ever remove. These persons may get on very well in their allotted part,
and even achieve distinction, while the insane
element is often cropping out in the shape of ex-
travagancies or irregularities of thought or action, which, according to the stand-point they are
viewed from, are regarded as gross eccentricity,
or undisciplined powers, or downright insanity.
For every manifestation of this kind they may
show no lack of plausible reasons, calculated to
mislead the superficial observer; but still the fact
remains that these traits, which are never witnessed in persons of well-balanced minds, are a
part of their habitual character. When persons
of this description possess a high order of intel-

lectual endowments, the unhealthy element often seems to impart force and piquancy to their mental manifestations, and thus increases the embarrassment touching the true character of their mental constitution. When the defect appears in the reflective powers, it is regarded as insanity by many who would give it a very different name were it confined to the emotions and feelings. But the man who goes through life creditably performing his part, though oscillating between the two states of excessive depression and excessive exhilaration, is as clearly under the influence of disease as if he believed in imaginary plots and conspiracies against his property or person. In neither case is he completely overborne by the force of the strange impression, but passes along, to all appearance, much like other men. Insane, in the popular acceptation, he certainly is not; but it is equally certain that his mind is not in a healthy condition. Lord Byron was one of the class in question, and the fact gives us a clue to the anomalies of his character. His mother was subject to violent outbreaks of passion, not unlike those often witnessed in the insane. On the paternal side his case was scarcely better. The loose principles, the wild and reckless conduct of his father, procured for him the nickname of " *Mad Jack Byron*"; and his grand-uncle, who killed his neigh-

bor in a duel, exhibited traits not very characteristic of a healthy mind. With such antecedents, it is not strange that he was subject to
wild impulses, violent passions, baseless prejudices, uncompromising selfishness, irregular mental activity. The morbid element in his nervous
system was also witnessed in the form of epilepsy, from which he suffered, more or less, during his whole life. The " vile melancholy " which
Dr. Johnson inherited from his father, and which,
to use his own expression, " made him mad all
his life, at least, not sober," never perverted the
exercise of his intellectual powers. He heard
the voice of his distant mother calling " Sam ";
he was bound to touch every post he passed in
the streets; he astonished people by his extraordinary singularities ; and much of his time was
spent in the depths of mental distress; yet the
march of his intellect, steady, uniform, and
measured, gave no token of confusion or weakness.

In common life this kind of mental dualism is
not unfrequent, though generally regarded as
anomalous and unaccountable, rather than the
result of an organic law. In some, the morbid
element, without affecting the keenness of the
intellect, intrudes itself on all occasions and
characterizes the ways and manners, the demeanor and deportment. Under the influence

3

of peculiarly adverse circumstances, they are liable to lose the unsteady balance between the antagonistic forces of their mental nature, to conduct as if unquestionably insane, and to be treated accordingly. Of such, the remark is always made by the world, which sees no nice distinctions, " If he is insane now, he was always insane." According as the one or the other phasis of their mind is exclusively regarded, they are accounted by some as always crazy, by others as uncommonly shrewd and capable.

In some persons the morbid element appears in the shape of insensibility to nice moral distinctions. Their perception of them at all seems to be the result of imitation rather than instinct. With them, circumstances determine everything as to the moral complexion of their career in life. Whether they leave behind them a reputation for flagrant selfishness, meanness, and dishonesty, or for a commendable prudence and judicious regard for self, — whether they always keep within the precincts of a decent respectability, or run into disreputable courses, — depends mostly on chance and fortune. This intimate association of the saint and the sinner in the same individual, common as it is, is a stumbling-block to moralists and legislators. The abnormal element is entirely overlooked, or rather, is confounded with that kind of moral depravity which comes from vicious training. The distinction is not always very easily made; for though sufficient light on this point may often be derived from the antecedents of the individuals, yet it is impossible, occasionally, to remove the obscurity in which it is involved. However this may be, it is a warrantable inference from the results of modern inquiry, that the class of cases is not a small one, where the person commits a criminal act, or falls into vicious habits, with a full knowledge of the nature and consequences of his conduct, and prompted, perhaps, by the ordinary inducements to vice, who, nevertheless, might have been a shining example of virtue, had the morbid element in his cerebral organism been left out. In our rough estimates of responsibility this goes for nothing, like the untoward influences of education; and it could not well be otherwise, though it cannot be denied that one element of moral responsibility, namely, the wish and the power to pursue the right and avoid the wrong, is greatly defective.

There is another phasis of cerebral defect not very unlike the last, which of late years has been occurring with increasing frequency, embarrassing our courts, confounding the wise and the simple, and overwhelming respectable families with shame and sorrow. With an intellect unwarped by the slightest excitement or delusion,

and with many moral traits, it may be, calculated
to please and to charm, its subjects are irresistibly impelled to some particular form of crime.
With more or less effort perhaps they strive
against it, and when they yield their conduct is
as much a mystery to themselves as to others.

From what has been stated, it may be inferred
that we are not yet acquainted with all the conditions of hereditary transmission, and therefore
we should not too readily be shaken in our belief of the general fact, by those incidents which
seem to indicate a violation of its known laws.
Among the lower animals, as well as the human
races, individuals of extraordinary excellence occasionally appear under circumstances which
render their appearance seemingly fortuitous.
They are neither preceded nor succeeded by individuals of remarkable endowments, and they
come and go like many other happy accidents of
nature that defy even a plausible explanation.
The parents of Shakespeare, of Milton, of Scott,
were indifferent persons, and their descendants
were scarcely distinguished from the multitude
around them. So too those heroes of the turf,
the Eclipses, the Highflyers, the Flying Childers,
stand alone, scarcely sharing their fame with
any of kindred blood. When this subject comes
to be fully understood, it will be seen that these
apparent anomalies result from the action of

laws as precise and inflexible as those by which the features of the child are assimilated to those of the parent. In regard to many of the phenomena of life, no one doubts that they are governed by laws, while no one undertakes to say what these laws are. For instance, the difference of sex, and the proportion in point of numbers existing between the two, we believe to be governed by laws, and none the less confidently, because they have completely eluded the researches of philosophers. Thus, while we are unable to account for the production of those isolated geniuses who have enlarged our conceptions of the human capacity, we are not obliged to abate one jot of our conviction, that, in a very great degree, the most remarkable endowments, wherever existing, are determined by the laws of hereditary transmission.

A not infrequent cause of mental deterioration is the intermarriage of blood relations. The great physiological law, that like produces like, depends upon this condition, that the parents shall not be nearly allied by blood. In the domestic animals, neglect of this condition is soon followed by deterioration, and if continued through several generations, the original good qualities of the breed disappear altogether. In man this effect is less obvious, parties often escaping any apparent penalty, even

when the law is violated in two successive generations. But it is common enough and severe
enough to render infractions of the law fearfully
hazardous. Its existence has been denied on
the strength of some limited statistics, but the
stern facts on the subject are too numerous to
be accidental, and it must be our own fault if
we do not heed the lesson which they teach.
Because the physical qualities of the parents are
occasionally too prominent and too well established to be materially vitiated by a single infringement of the law, and the first impression
is not enforced and reduplicated by repetitions
of the infringement, men are disposed to believe
that they have committed no transgression!

Within a few years past, the physiological
effects upon the offspring, of marriages in con-
sanguinity have been carefully investigated by
Devay, Perrin, Menière, and others, in France,
and Bemiss and Howe in this country. These
inquiries show, among these effects, an extraordinary proportion of disease and imperfection
in the shape of insanity, idiocy, epilepsy, blind-
ness, deaf-mutism, and sterility. From 24 to 30
per cent. of all the pupils in the institutions of
France for deaf mutes are the offspring of such
marriages, and many of them left a deaf mute
brother or sister at home. Dr. Howe collected the
statistics of seventeen marriages in consanguin-

ity, from which it appears that of the ninety-five children which proceeded from them, forty-four were idiots, twelve scrofulous and delicate, one deaf, and one a dwarf. Dr. Bemiss has collated the results of eight hundred and thirty-three consanguineous marriages, reported by himself and others, from which proceeded thirty-nine hundred and forty-two children. Of these, one hundred and forty-five were deaf mutes, eighty-five blind, three hundred and eight idiotic, thirty-eight insane, sixty epileptic, three hundred scrofulous, ninety-eight deformed, and one hundred defective in one way or another.

In persons of a feeble capacity, and especially such as have some tendency to disease, the evil in question is more likely to follow ; and cases of this kind 'are not rare in the experience of those much conversant with mental disorders. The operation of the law may be always witnessed in families which, for one reason or another, have formed their matrimonial alliances within themselves for many generations. I could mention a community where, for the purpose of keeping property together, marriages between near relations have been frequent, in which the remarkable prevalence of insanity and other disorders and imperfections supposed to be incident to such connections, has arrested the attention of the most superficial observers. Many of my readers, no doubt, can call to mind similar cases. In the royal houses of Spain, Portugal, and Austria, this is the worm that gnawed at the root of their strength, and brought on debility and decay. The elder members were the marked men of their times, distinguished by their physical and mental endowments. In almost every marriage among their descendants the parties had more or less of common blood, and the result is plainly written in the history of Europe during the last hundred years.

The remarkable difference exhibited by communities not very different in other respects, in the amount of insanity and other mental infirmities, exemplifies another phasis of cerebral deterioration. It may be doubted whether, in this country even, where the mingling of common blood in the matrimonial connection is more frequent than is generally supposed, any other agency whatever has had more to do with the prevalence of insanity and idiocy than this. In many of our small, secluded towns, one has only to cast his eye over the list of voters suspended in the bar-room of the tavern, or by the church-door, to see how large a proportion of the people is embraced in a few leading names seldom met with anywhere else. This naturally implies a good deal of intermarriage, and an extensive infusion of common blood.

The fact furnishes a clew to an explanation of another order of facts which have caused some speculation both here and abroad. The general impression has been that mental disease is more rife in commercial and manufacturing communities, where reverses are more common and the mind is subjected to a greater tension, than in agricultural communities, where life flows on in a more uniform current. The theory is plausible, but not sustained by facts. The circumstances supposed have much to do, no doubt, with determining the mental condition of the people, but a little inquiry will show us that there is another agent more potent than these, and one whose power is more felt in the country than in populous cities and mushroom villages. The statistics of insanity in Massachusetts, collected in 1854, by Dr. Edward Jarvis, by order of the Legislature, show very clearly the absence of any connection between the disease and the pursuits of the people. Looking over the returns from the counties of Essex, Middlesex, Worcester, and Suffolk, we find that two of them have more, and two less than the average amount of insanity in the whole State; and yet, in point of mental stir and excitement, they are, probably, very nearly alike. The rural counties show the same want of uniformity; while, taken together, they can claim no advantage in regard to the point in question over the maritime counties. The mountain breezes of Berkshire and the quiet pursuits of its people seem to be no more conducive to mental integrity than the chilling winds of Essex, Suffolk, and Plymouth, and the changing fortunes of their people. It also appears that the principal manufacturing places, Lowell, Lawrence, Worcester, Lynn, Taunton, Fall River, Waltham, Milford, Palmer, Fitchburg, and Blackstone, with an aggregate population of 154,975, have 221 insane persons, or 1 in 701 ; whereas in the counties of Berkshire, Hampshire, and Franklin, with a population of 122,730, less changeable than any other in the State, we find 472 insane persons, or 1 in 258. No State in the Union, probably, has so large a proportion of insanity as Massachusetts, and no other has so large a proportion of old communities. A similar class of facts was observed by Her Majesty's commissioners appointed in 1855 to inquire into the state of lunatic asylums in Scotland. They say in their Report, that " in those counties where thought most stagnates, a large proportion of the cases of mental disease is due to congenital causes. The population, unaffected by extraneous influences, intermarry among themselves, and the hereditary taint which is thus engendered, shows itself unmistakably in the large

proportion of idiots and imbeciles." They compare the statistics of mental disease in the remote counties with those of the southern counties, " where the mental powers have been more
called into action, and intermarriage is less frequent, and the result is, that a Highland population contains more than three times the number
of congenital cases of mental disease found in
an equal Lowland population; and that the
difference becomes much greater if the comparison be confined to single counties of the two
series." Here the cause of the disproportion is
distinctly alleged, and it seems to be a fair conclusion that there is a more potent agency in
the production of mental disease than the in-
dustrial pursuits of the people, — one which
vitiates the physical qualities of the race in
the very germs of life. If this view is correct,
it explains a fact in the history of mental disease, which has always been a matter of surprise. I refer to the large number of cases'
which cannot be attributed to any particular
cause or concurrence of causes. The disease
takes place as if it were the natural result of
the development of the individual, — the operation, it may be, of that great organic law which
forbids the union of offspring from a common
stock, by the penalty of disease and deterioration.

Another potent agency in vitiating the quality of the brain is habitual intemperance, and the effect is far oftener witnessed in the offspring than in the drunkard himself. His habits may induce an attack of insanity, where the predisposition exists; but he generally escapes with nothing worse than the loss of some of his natural vigor and hardihood of mind. In the offspring, however, on whom the consequences of the parental vice may be visited, to the third if not the fourth generation, the cerebral disorder may take the form of intemperance, or idiocy, or insanity, or vicious habits, or impulses to crime, or some minor mental obliquities.

The frequency with which intemperance is witnessed, both in parent and child, has come to be regarded not as a matter of accident merely, but as the result of hereditary cerebral defect. There have been cases enough the circumstances of which excluded the influence of vicious example and training, and rendered no other explanation possible but this. The reader will, no doubt, readily recur to examples of the saddest kind that have fallen under his own observation.

As a cause of idiocy in the next succeeding generation, the potency of gross intemperance has been placed beyond a doubt. Dr. S. G. Howe, who once thoroughly investigated the antecedents of a great many cases of idiocy, came to the conclusion that, "directly or indirectly, alcohol is productive of a great proportion of the idiocy which now burdens the Commonwealth of Massachusetts." *

The transmitted effect of intemperance may also appear in the form of a propensity to vicious courses, or a dulness of moral perception, or irresistible impulses to crime. One child may exhibit one or more of these traits, and another may be insane or idiotic, the former no less than the latter manifesting the legitimate effects of the parent's vice. The inmates of our penitentiaries, whose history is thoroughly known, present many examples of the operation of this pathological law.

There is this curious feature of the deteriorating influence of intemperance, that its primary effect is not always persistent, but may be removed by removing the cause. In the Report of the hospital at Columbus, Ohio, for 1861, the physician, Dr. Hills, says of one of his patients, that his father, in the first part of his married life, was strictly temperate, "and had four children, all yet remaining healthy and sound. From reverses of fortune, he became discouraged and intemperate for some years, having in

* Report made to the Legislature of Massachusetts on Idiocy, p. 83.

this period four children, two of whom we had now received into the asylum ; a third one was idiotic, and the fourth epileptic. He then reformed in habits, had three more children, all now grown to maturity, and to this period remaining sound and healthy." Another similar case follows. An intemperate parent had four children, two of whom became insane, one was an idiot, and the fourth died young, in fits. Four children born previous to the period of intemperance, and two after the parent's reformation, are all sound and healthy.

Another very important condition requisite to the highest degree of mental health and vigor is that of a healthy, vigorous body. There are people in the world, even in this age of enlightenment, who believe, or act as if they believed, that there is no necessary connection between these two things. In all matters of education and hygiene, they practically regard the mind as perfectly independent of the body. Indeed, they seem to look upon bodily imperfections as actually favorable to mental activity and vigor, for the same reason, I suppose, that the blind are known to acquire uncommon acuteness of hearing and touch. It has been one of the traditionary customs of our country, not entirely extinct yet, to select from the sons of the family the feeble, sickly youth, apparently incapable of

earning his living by the sweat of his brow, to
be the favored recipient of an education that will
fit him to live by his wits. To this custom, apparently, one of our greatest men — great at the
bar, in the senate, in the cabinet — was indebted
for that change of destiny which produced such
magnificent results, though in his case there was
less reason for the change than was apprehend-
ed. We meet with instances, no doubt, that
seem to support the popular view — of feeble,
perhaps sickly, bodies associated with strong and
capacious minds. Such cases, however, are but
exceptions to the general rule, and we never can
be sure that the mental efficiency would not
have been considerably increased had the physical condition been of a healthier character. Men
of superior cultivation and energy of will may
rise above the enervating influence of bodily infirmity, and, though scarcely a day exempt from
pain, move along in their accustomed course,
challenging the admiration of the world by the
steadiness of their application and the brilliancy
of their achievements.

No one can be insensible to the moral grandeur of such triumphs of mind over matter, as
were exemplified in Pascal, who, while tortured
with infirmities that embittered his existence, and
hallucinations that destroyed his peace of mind,
launched upon the world that imperishable model

of wit, raillery, and eloquence, the Provincial
Letters; in Cowper, surrounded nearly all his
life by clouds and darkness, but achieving an
honorable place in the literature of his country;
in Robert Hall, while writing those sermons
which electrified the public mind of England, in
the intervals between paroxysms of the severest
bodily anguish; in Channing, never faltering in
his chosen work of elevating the purposes and
sentiments of his age, though under the unceasing pressure of ill-health, if not positive pain.
Seldom, however, is bodily ailment met by such
indomitable power of resistance. Its usual effect, especially in persons of moderate capacity,
is to embarrass the action of the mind, to enfeeble
its conceptions, to diminish its power of application, to quench its aspirations, and shut out
the blessed sunshine which never entirely ceases
to gild the prospects of the mortal who rejoices
in the buoyant sensations of sound health. In
those who are habitually ailing, all the surplus
energy is needed to meet the demands of the
suffering organs. Starting from the seat of the
disease, a host of abnormal impressions crowd
on the mind, distracting its attention from all
higher contemplations, and concentrating its
thoughts and cares and interests upon the present moment. In most men, neither philosophy
nor religion can place the mind at ease and

ready for intellectual effort, when consumption
is wasting the vital energies, or dyspepsia is
sharpening the sensibility of every nerve, or
hypochondria is filling the soul with dismal apprehensions. In such circumstances the largest
intellect may be engrossed with trifles, and the
most benevolent heart may overflow with gall
and bitterness. The pleasurable emotions that
arise from mental occupation are replaced by
pain or *ennui*; the ordinary inducements to effort utterly fail; social intercourse, even, loses its
charms, and life itself may become a cheerless
waste in which man delighteth not, nor woman
neither. Johnson has touchingly described —
probably from experience — the condition of a
" man of an active and elevated mind, laboring
under the weight of a distempered body." " The
time of such a man," he says, " fumes away in
projects and in hope, and the day of action
never comes. He lies down delighted with the
thoughts of to-morrow, pleases his ambition with
the fame he shall acquire, or his benevolence
with the good he shall confer: but in the night,
the skies are overcast, the temperature of the
air is changed ; he awakes in languor, impatience, and distraction ; and has no longer any
wish but for ease, nor any attention but to mis-
ery." With reason, then, did an eminent writer
say, " The heir of a sound constitution has no

4

right to regret the absence of any other patri-
mony. A man who has derived from the immediate authors of his being vigorous and un-
tainted stamina of mind as well as of body,
enters upon the world with a sufficient foundation and ample materials for happiness." *

Very few of those men who have achieved
great intellectual renown, suffered much from
ill-health. The distinguished names in English
literature, for instance, belonged for the most
part to sound, strong, healthy men; and it was
by reason of their being sound, strong, and
healthy, that they accomplished what they did.
Newton went through his course of mathemat-
ical investigation, undisturbed by a single day
of sickness; and if subsequently, under excessive application and loss of sleep, his majestic
intellect passed under a cloud, it shortly emerged
from it in all its original brightness. Bacon, by
means of a robust and hardy constitution, was
able, in addition to professional duties which
would have been quite enough for most men, to
engage in a course of philosophical inquiry that
laid anew the very foundations of human knowledge. That nice discernment of character which
has made Shakespeare the poet of all times and
of all people, could have sprung only from perceptions never clouded nor distorted by the mor-

* Dr. Reid; *Hypochondriacal and other Nervous Affections.*

bid influences of poor health.   Burke, who, from first to last, in one way or another, accomplished an amount and a kind of intellectual effort that have placed him in the foremost rank of great men, scarcely lost a day by sickness, until the period of his breaking up.   Walter Scott was sustained in his career, than which the annals of literature can show none more brilliant, by the energies of a frame well-fitted by nature, and trained by daily habits of exercise and recrea- tion, for remarkable power of endurance.

It may be also said of men engaged in the active business of life, that the highest degree of health is necessary to insure the most complete and satisfactory result.   Countless examples might be adduced from among those whose names are written on the page of history, to show how much they were indebted for their distinction to good health.   The two great war- riors of our age, for instance, owed their success, not more to extraordinary mental abilities than to the vigor of their bodily powers, which sup- ported those abilities under the severest toil and sacrifice.   The rest and recreation which Wel- lington craved amid the fatigues of the camp was to follow the hounds; and, after spending the day in earnestly watching the movements of a hostile army, he could retire to his tent and write a masterly memoir on the project of estab-

lishing a national bank in Portugal. The Her-
culean labors of Napoleon in the closet as well
as the field, in bringing the forces of nature and
the wills of men into his marvellous combinations, and personally directing the affairs of an
immense empire, required an iron frame and
nerves beyond the reach of fatigue. Once he
suffered from the frailties of the flesh, and on
that occasion he met his first decisive check.
On the fruitless field of Borodino, where his fate
depended upon the result, he remained far in the
rear, dull and dejected, learning the progress of
the battle without interest or emotion. He was
exhausted by fatigue and anxiety, he had taken
a severe cold over night, and on that day he had
an attack of an eminently painful disease. In
short, in any sphere of life where mental activity
is required, the highest measure of success can
seldom be expected by those who suffer from
habitual infirmity of body. The world is full
of melancholy illustrations of this position. The
genius that has been nipped in the bud, the talents that have been paralyzed, the plans that
have been defeated, the hopes that have been
destroyed, by disordered health, — who can estimate their amount! The youth who escapes
from the perils of early life with the powers of
his constitution unimpaired, succumbs in early
manhood, just as society is reckoning upon a

brilliant career of usefulness and distinction; and the full-grown adult, who has given the world assurance of a man, is cut down in a green old age, perhaps in the midst of unfinished performances.

The amount of mental power which has thus been destroyed is infinitely greater, no doubt, than that which has been suffered to work out its destined purpose, enforced by the sustaining influences of sound health. Although the rate of mortality has been steadily declining, yet it is no less true that disease and infirmity were never more prevalent in the civilized world than at the present day. Few, indeed, but medical men, are aware of the appalling magnitude of the evil. Those who are aware of it seem to be led by its very magnitude to believe that it is something inevitable, a part of the ordinary routine of nature; as if infirmity and disease were the rule and good health the exception. Indeed, there is much reason for such a belief. Who can find among his acquaintances a single family every member of which has enjoyed uninterrupted health for half a dozen years together? It was not always so. The time has been when men, ay, and women, after weathering the usual diseases of childhood, passed on to a ripe old age, scarcely making the acquaintance of the phy-

sician, and meeting no token of mortality more
significant than an occasional cold, or, possibly,
an attack of fever. Those much-enduring men
and women who encountered the privations of
the colonial times have been succeeded by a
race incapable of their toil and exposure, whom
the winds of heaven cannot visit too roughly
without leaving behind the seeds of dissolution.
It would be inconsistent with my present purpose to inquire how it happens that a people
suffering as little as any the evils incident to the
extremes of social condition, should nevertheless
be characteristically prone to every form of mental and bodily ailment, but the fact is sufficiently
important to deserve a thorough investigation.
I can notice it only as one among the most
efficient causes of insanity in this country; and
so well is this fact recognized by those who have
charge of hospitals for the insane, that wherever
the causes of the disease are given, *ill-health*
predominates over every other in the number of
its victims. By far the larger portion is contributed by the female sex, whose ill-health generally implies a state of nervous exhaustion and
enfeeblement produced by excessive labor and
trial, in a constitution endowed by nature with
little power of endurance. Of course, the evil
is chiefly confined to those classes of women
whose duties require a considerable amount of

hard work, or excessive application to the lighter forms of labor. In the married state, the laudable ambition of showing a house and family distinguished by all the indications of good management, induces them to labor beyond their strength, while little or nothing is done towards restoring it by suitable relaxation. The cares of an increasing family, without increasing pecuniary means, seem to forbid the slightest rest from the daily routine of toil; their duties are all within doors, in overheated apartments, while a certain regard for appearances, and a perpetual straining after a higher social sphere, give rise to an uneasy, if not repining state of mind. At last, the appetite fails, the nervous system becomes irritable under the slightest impression, the sleep is diminished, the flesh reduced, and the mind depressed by unaccountable gloom and apprehension. From this to unequivocal insanity, the transition is only a matter of time. With the corresponding classes of the old world, it is all very different. They work hard and fare hard, it is true; but they start with a stronger constitution; they are much in the open air; they live on plain food; and move in a social sphere that bounds all their wishes and aspirations.

Besides an effect so severe and striking as that of actual disease, it can scarcely be questioned that an evil so prevalent and powerful as this exerts considerable influence on the mental character of the people. Such, I believe to be the case, for the proofs of it are too many and too strong to escape the intelligent observer. We may see one of them in the increasing fondness for light reading, especially for such as is addressed to the emotions and passions. It is lamentable how many persons capable of better things read only for amusement, with no wish to gain information, or enjoy the higher charms of literature. They share the opinion of the poet Gray, who could conceive of no greater luxury, he said, than to "lie on a sofa all day and read eternal new novels of Marivaux and Crebillon." This wretched taste is confined to no particular class. Once, the yellow-covered literature, as it is called, was to be found only on railroads and steamboats, and, in corporal dimensions, seldom exceeded the modest limits of a pamphlet. Within a few years it has greatly enlarged its pretensions, and become an institution of the times. It has swelled into the more respectable dimensions of the duodecimo and octavo; it rejoices in all the attractions which the printer and engraver can give it; it forms the staple of the circulating library; it has secured a place upon the centre-table; and claims a notice from the reviews. The aim of this class

of books is to kindle strange emotions; they
display the morbid anatomy of the passions;
and their tendency is to loosen the hold of the
mind on eternal principles and allow it to wander on in its dim and perilous way, with no better guide than the allurements of sense or the
humors of the time. It remains to be explained
why it is that literature, whose proper function
is to strengthen the intellectual faculties, to
quicken the moral perceptions, to widen the field
of sympathy, to establish the supremacy of the
higher sentiments, should be made, in this our
day and generation, to serve a very different
purpose,—to stimulate a prurient imagination,
to bring the aspirations and sympathies within
the circle of an intense selfishness, and substi-
tute a sickly sentimentality for those sharp
moral distinctions that spring from true, practical, healthy views of life. Some may think it
a fanciful speculation to suppose that the characteristic traits of the popular literature may be
fairly attributed to our extraordinary proneness
to ill-health. But we instinctively speak of the
prevalent taste as *unhealthy,* as if it were the only
epithet that could suitably express its character,
and we certainly cannot explain it on any other
hypothesis. Considering the increase of knowledge and refinement, and the host of examples
of whatever is pure and graceful and sublime in

English literature, we might have reasonably
expected a different result.   While the cause remains we shall continue to witness the effect.
While so large a portion of our people labor
under a feverish pulse, a disturbed digestion,
and irritable nerves, there will be, as a natural
consequence, this craving for an intense and exciting literature; and even here we have no exception to the prevalent law of demand and
supply.

Good health and freedom from morbid tendencies, important as they certainly are, are not the
only physical qualities necessary to the attainment of the highest degree of mental efficiency.
The secret of many a man's greatness may be
found, not in remarkable endowments of mind,
but in a bodily constitution possessing extraordinary powers of endurance.   This it is, and
this only, which sustains the industry, the patience, the indomitable perseverance, indispensable to the highest success in many a distinguished career.   Some men there are — their
number, alas, is small — upon whom no amount
of mental labor makes any impression, and
though not particularly careful of themselves,
they prove to be superior to all the ills of mortality.   No stretch of attention can weary them,
no degree of application can obscure the clear-
ness of their conceptions, and no amount of

taskwork can exceed the limits of their endurance. Without recreation and with stinted rest, they work on, scarcely conscious of fatigue, and always ready for fresh toil. The same tasks which would leave other men exhausted and spiritless, seem to impart to them additional vigor and elasticity. Year after year they pursue the same round of unceasing labor, and while everybody is predicting premature decay, they leave the wrecks of their contemporaries behind and flourish on to a ripe old age. They are to be found among the generals who have pursued an unbroken career of victory; among the statesmen who have controlled the policy of nations; among the mechanics and engineers whose conceptions embodied in wood and iron have shaped the destiny of the age. It is this marvellous constitution alone which makes all the difference between men like Wellington, Washington, Scott, Franklin, Palmerston, Lyndhurst, Brougham, Cuvier, Stephenson, and the countless host who leave behind them merely the reputation of promising men prematurely struck down. We have no reason to believe that the human constitution is normally inferior, in point of endurance, to that of the brutes; and yet with all the advantages of reason, and all our pride of race, we are far behind them all in this respect. In civilized nations, more than one

third of the race perish within five years after
birth; and only one in five or six reaches the
appointed term of human life,—threescore years
and ten. In view of these facts, men are inclined to derive consolation from the idea, that
these physical deficiencies are more than coun-
terbalanced by the excellence of our mental
stamina; and while the lungs are nourishing
the seeds of consumption, and the stomach is
destined to fall an easy prey to dyspepsia, and
the nerves are tortured, even from the cradle,
with anomalous ills, we flatter ourselves that
the brain is beyond the reach of their noxious
influences, and in the undisturbed possession of
its normal powers!

It may possibly be feared by those worthy
people who find themselves beyond their depth
the moment they leave the shore of time-honor-
ed opinions, that, in attributing so much as we
have thus far to merely organic conditions — in
making the mental so dependent on the physical
— we thereby weaken the foundations of all moral
distinction.   As this apprehension may cause
some distrust of the soundness of our principles,
and so far impair the force of their hygienic application, it may be well to show how little support the popular views on this subject derive
from true science and sound common sense.

While people clearly recognize the infinite di-

versity of intellectual gifts, and would no more
expect the fruits of genius and talent from them
who had been denied by nature the slightest
portion of either, than we should grapes from
thorns or figs from thistles, they are in the habit
of believing that, for all practical purposes, the
moral endowments of men are equal. Not exactly that they are equally benevolent, equally
honest, equally true to the right and the good,
but that they might be if they chose. Misled by
the fallacies which lurk under the specious terms,
free will, free agency, they reach the conclusion
that all men are equally responsible for their deviations from the line of moral rectitude. They
never would think of saying to men, " Here is
poetry, here is philosophy, here is art; you have
the capacity to excel in either ; take your choice,
and the world will hold you responsible for the
result;" yet they do not see the absurdity of
saying, " Do good or do evil; be a saint or a
sinner, a blessing or a curse to your race; you
are a free agent, take your choice, and be rewarded or punished accordingly." But those
cabalistic words, *free will, free agency*, which
have been used, time out of mind, to dispel the
difficulties of human responsibility, have now
lost their force, and we are obliged to resort for
light to the results of modern inquiry.

In the *moral sense* or *faculty*, it is easy to recognize two different elements, viz. the power to discern the distinction between right and wrong, virtue and vice, the honest and the base, and the disposition to pursue the one and avoid the other. These elements, like those of the intellect, are unequally developed in different men, which inequality may be either congenital, or produced in after life, by moral or physical causes. And thus though a person may act with perfect freedom of will, unconscious of any irresistible bias, yet it is obvious that his conduct is actually governed more by these variable conditions of his moral nature, than by any abstract notions formed by the intellect. In our ordinary judgments of men, as well as in those severer judgments that proceed from legal tribunals, the former are generally left out of the account; but it cannot be supposed that, in determining the measure of responsibility, they are entirely without their weight, in the mind of the Sovereign Judge and Disposer. Now, then, starting from the unquestioned fact that the brain is the material instrument of the mind, we are led to the inevitable conclusion that its physical condition must modify more or less its mental manifestations, moral as well as intellectual. To deny so plain a proposition would be equivalent to denying that the quality of the instrument or organ can affect the quality of the result which it was intended to produce, — to denying, in fact, that the quality of the music depends, in any degree, on the excellence of the instrument as well as the skill of the musician. We almost instinctively recognize the connection between a large and well-proportioned head and great mental powers ; between the diminutive head and a very limited development of mind. In the various races of men, the dullest observer may see that the cerebral indicates very exactly the mental development; and the sculptor or painter who should disregard these relations would be considered stupid enough to be beyond the reach of censure. It follows, therefore, that the quality of the brain as affected by breeding, whereby a high or a low degree of organic excellence is made permanent, by being persistently transmitted through several generations, or by the influence of morbid action in itself or in other organs of the body, must determine, in a great degree, the moral as well as the intellectual character of each individual man. It is said in the common form of speech, that a person is good or bad, because he *chooses* to be the one or the other ; and it is all very true, and sufficient, perhaps, for our rough estimates of responsibility, but it does not answer the essential question, What determines the choice ? In the considerations here presented, and in these only, is to be found a satisfactory answer to this question.

The doctrine here put forth has been so admirably unfolded by a popular writer, the secret of whose success consists not more in the force and humor of his conceptions than in the sound philosophy which pervades his views of moral and social questions, that I cannot forbear to make a liberal quotation. " Ministers talk about the human will as if it stood on a high look-out, with plenty of light and elbow-room reaching to the horizon. Doctors are constantly noticing how it is tied up and darkened by inferior organization, by disease, and all sorts of crowding interferences, until they get to look upon Hottentots and Indians — and a good many of their own race — as a kind of self-conscious blood-clocks, with very limited power of self-determination. That's the tendency, I say, of a doctor's experience. But the people to whom they address their statements of the results of their observation belong to the thinking class of the highest races, and they are conscious of a great deal of liberty of will. So in the face of the fact that civilization with all its offers has proved a dead failure with the aboriginal races of this country, — on the whole, I say, a dead failure, — they talk as if they knew from their own will all about that of a Digger Indian. . . .

We see all kinds of monomania and insanity. We learn from them to recognize all sorts of queer tendencies in minds supposed to be sane, so that we have nothing but compassion for a large class of persons condemned as sinners by theologians, but considered by us as invalids. We have constant reasons for noticing the transmission of qualities from parents to offspring, and we find it hard to hold a child accountable in any moral point of view for inherited bad temper, or tendency to drunkenness, — as hard as we should to blame him for inheriting gout or asthma." *

* *Elsie Venner*, ii. 115.

5

CHAPTER II.

MENTAL HYGIENE AS AFFECTED BY PHYSICAL IN-
FLUENCES.

AMONG the physical agents that affect the
vigor of the mind, none is more worthy of our
attention than the air which we breathe, especially as its importance in this respect is not
sufficiently considered. Nobody denies that bad
air is unwholesome, but most people suppose
that the mischief is confined to the organs of
respiration. The physiologist knows, however,
that, much as these organs unquestionably suffer from bad air, the brain, on the whole, suffers
more. If the blood which is sent from the lungs
to the rest of the system is imperfectly oxygen-
ated, no organ feels it more than the brain. It
needs no argument better than one's own sensations, to prove that in the open air, where we
may inhale the breezes of heaven without let or
hindrance, we experience, in the highest degree,
its refreshing and invigorating influence. So
susceptible is the brain of aerial changes that
can only be manifested to it through the blood,
that, were we deprived of every sense, we should

have no difficulty in distinguishing between the
air of a room and the air of the open sky.

Besides the merely pleasurable sensation derived from pure air, there is also a positive influence exerted by it on the mental movements.
The thoughts succeed one another more rapidly, the conceptions are clearer, the mental activity can be longer maintained, and a certain
feeling of buoyancy, if not exhilaration, pervades
the whole mental condition. In a school, or
hospital, or any other considerable assembly of
people, the purity of the air may be pretty accu-
rately measured by the amount of cheerfulness,
activity, and lively interest which pervades it.
And yet so little do people think or care about
this subject, that, under existing arrangements,
there are very few who do not, every day of their
lives, inspire more or less highly vitiated air. In
the school-room, where many a youth spends a
large portion of his early life, the same air is
generally breathed over and over again ; and the
only attempt which modern ingenuity has devised, or modern thrift has allowed, for remedy-
ing the evil, consists in some trumpery contriv-
ance whose operation depends on the state of the
external atmosphere. In churches, in lecture-
rooms, in court-rooms, and ball-rooms, where people are wont to congregate, we have the same
evil, and perhaps the same abortive attempt to

relieve it. In thousands of shops and counting-
rooms the air is vitiated, for several months in
the year, by coming in contact with red-hot
iron, and often, by carbonic acid gas escaping
from a leaky apparatus. But being early habit-
uated to this kind of air, the greater part of our
people grow up with their native sense of atmospherical purity completely perverted. Even
men whose education has made them acquainted with the laws of the animal economy,
and whose avocations, it might be supposed,
would leave them ample opportunity to care
for their health, seem to be as regardless of
good air as any others.

The effect of vitiated air on the animal economy is not often very perceptible immediately.
The scholar recites his lessons, the merchant toils
over his ledger, the minister, the lecturer, the
judge, each performs his part, without growing
black in the face, or falling down in a state of
asphyxia. Most of them are not aware of having been under any noxious influence. A gentleman who, for many years, sat upon the Supreme Bench of Massachusetts, which he hon-
ored by his learning and integrity, and who, in
the course of his life, had probably inspired more
bad air than any other professional man of his
time, used to express his surprise that so much
was said about pure air and bad air, because it

seemed to be all alike to him. But the mischief is no less serious because its consequences are not immediately perceptible, any more than many other improprieties in our modes of living. Much of the ill-health to which we have already adverted arises probably from this source. But often the immediate effect is obvious to the vigilant observer. The natural elasticity of the mind, which enables it, easily and promptly, to keep to its work, is impaired, and its operations are maintained by a dogged effort of the will. The jaded, wearisome feeling is prolonged into the intervals of rest, and, much of the time, the individual is conscious that he has a brain, more by the discomfort it occasions than by those pleasurable emotions that mark its perfectly healthy condition.

It is a fact of considerable importance to the nervous invalid, that, besides the matter of temperature, the external atmosphere is not the same at all times and in all places. Here it may be invigorating and bracing, filling the mind with energy and hope. There it makes every exertion a burden, and produces irresistible lassitude and listlessness. During the prevalence of the sirocco-wind in Malta, Sicily, and the south of Italy, there is observed to be a great increase of irritability and excitement, and nervous disease is more readily developed where the predisposi-

tion exists. The damp winds of **La Plata** produce a general lassitude and relaxation, accompanied by remarkable irritability and ill-humor.
It is a common thing for men among the better
classes to shut themselves up in their houses
during its continuance, and lay aside all business
until it has passed, while among the lower
classes cases of quarrelling and bloodshed are
more frequent. Everything is disarranged, and
everybody lays the fault to one source : " It is
the North wind, Señor."

" In some conditions of nervous disorder," says
a contemporary writer, "the slightest meteoro-
logical changes give rise to singular alternations
of despondency, despair, hope and joy, so completely does the mind succumb to physical influences. I have known a person subject to attacks of suicidal melancholia during the prevalence of a cold, blighting, depressing east wind,
who appeared happy, contented, and free from
all desire to injure himself under other and
more congenial conditions of the atmosphere.
An Italian artist never could reside a winter in
England without the distressing idea of self-destruction repeatedly suggesting itself to his morbidly depressed mind. I have known natives
cf France, accustomed from early life to the
buoyant air and light azure sky of that country,
sink into profound states of mental despon-

dency, if compelled to reside many weeks in London during the earlier portion of the winter season." *

The remarkable nervous excitability of our own people, indicated by restlessness, impulsiveness, impetuous and boisterous movement, probably arises from some quality of our climate. Certainly, there can be no doubt respecting the trait itself. From early childhood to mature decline, it is ever apparent, whether in the noise and rattle of the one, or the ardent, eager, insatiable spirit of the other. It is strikingly manifested in the insanity of this country, as compared with that of others. The most superficial observer does not fail to notice it in passing through the galleries of American and European hospitals for the insane. In the former, especially those of the Northern and Eastern States, more excitement will meet his notice in a single visit, than he will see in the latter, particularly the English, in a whole week or month. And yet this excitability is but little less apparent in the Germans, Irish, and English, who abound in our hospitals, than in the native Americans. Such facts should be duly considered by nervous invalids in deciding upon a change of climate, in order that the step may meet the requirements of their case.

* Winslow. *Obscure Diseases of the Mind*, p. 194.

To obtain the highest degree of mental vigor, we require suitable habits of bodily exercise. Indolence, or sedentary employment, is no less prejudicial to the health of the mind than to that of the body. And yet no class of men is more heedless of the fact than that which is engaged in mental occupations. The ministers, the lawyers, the employés in banks and counting-rooms, who shorten their days in consequence of such neglect, cannot be numbered. They depend upon their brain, as the day-laborer does upon his spade and pick, but treat it as if it were a machine designed, unlike all other machines of human construction, to run indefinitely, without repair, without even the slightest attention. " Other men look to their tools," says Burton; " a painter will wash his pencils ; a smith will look to his hammer, anvil, and forge; a husbandman will mend his plough-irons, and grind his hatchet if it be dull; a falconer or huntsman will have an especial care of his hawks, hounds, horses, and dogs ; a musician will string and unstring his lute ; only scholars neglect that instrument (their brain and spirits I mean) which they daily use, and by which they range over all the world, and which by much study is consumed."

To this as well as all other hygienic rules, there are, no doubt, some exceptions, and the

latter, unfortunately, are often regarded more
than the former. The literary or professional
man spends the greater part of the day in mental occupation, almost losing the use of his
muscles for want of practice. Blessed with a
native hardihood of constitution, he lives to a
ripe old age, and people wonder and admire at
the amount of work he has accomplished, and
hold him up, perhaps, as an example to be imitated. Another counts money, or posts books,
through the livelong day, with no other exercise
than a walk once or twice a day, between his
house and his office, and he too seems to thrive
upon it. All this may be so. Indeed, there is
no habit among those most generally regarded
as injurious to health, which may not be observed occasionally in connection with a high
degree of health. Still, the general rule is no
less true, nor less important. Activity is the
law of our being, imposed upon every organ of
the body. Absolute rest, except that required
by toil, nature abhors as she does a vacuum.
Instead of marking only exceptional cases, or
being curious as to the reasons for this or that
arrangement, it is better to recognize the law
and endeavor to comply with it. I repeat it,
that men whose pursuits require considerable
mental application, for several hours of the day,
cannot reasonably expect the highest degree of

mental vigor, without suitable habits of exercise.
Without entering into any elaborate investigation of its effects, it is enough here to say, that
it seems to be required in order to complete the
changes which the blood undergoes while passing through the lungs and skin, and by means
of which it supplies the necessary waste of material in the brain produced by excessive mental
application. In persons whose occupations are
merely sedentary, and who have little occasion
to think, this want of exercise is sufficiently mischievous, but when, in connection with sedentary habits, there is also much mental activity,
the mischief is greatly increased.

Even those who recognize the importance of
muscular exercise, and determine not to neglect
it altogether, are apt to take it very much as
they take physic, or perform any other disagreeable duty. They take a solitary walk or
ride, perhaps frequently and regularly while the
fit lasts, but improve the opportunity of being
more intent than usual on their customary
thoughts; and if, for the same purpose, they
hurry off every year or two to a watering-place,
or join the rush of a cheap excursion, their
minds are, all the while, away among the familiar scenes of business, and they long for the
moment which will terminate their unwelcome
absence. When fairly through with it, they feel

that they have laid up a supererogatory stock of health, sufficient for any present if not future contingency. Yet these persons would smile at the idea of swallowing, at one sitting, food enough to supply the calls of hunger for a week.

What is especially needed among us is a more prevalent and more practical conviction of the importance of physical exercise as a habit of life, — to be practised, not from a sense of duty, but because it is instinctively demanded by the necessities of our nature, and is a source of pleasurable sensations. We would do well to imitate the English in this respect, with whom the habit of daily exercise has become to a great extent an institution of society. Among the intelligent classes, few will be found who do not recognize and provide for this, as for other wants of nature. The English nobility, in spite of the indulgences which their position and means enable them to enjoy, are a long-lived race ; and it is because no class of people in the world spend a larger portion of their time engaged in exercise in the open air. The passion for field-sports is not confined to them, but prevails to an extent almost incredible to us, with whom it is barely respectable. And they whose avocations do not permit a habit of daily exercise, make up for it in some measure, by an an-

nual vacation, when work is abandoned for recreation and physical activity. The trader turns
his back upon the counter, the doctor abandons
his patients, the lawyer flies from the conflicts of
the bar — each and all determined to repair by
a month or two of sport or pleasure, the wear
and tear of the rest of the year.

The radical fault in our modes of exercise is
that they are unaccompanied by agreeable mental impressions. The mind is not diverted from
its usual channels while the muscles are in activity, and thus the whole affair becomes the
hardest description of work, resulting in fatigue
both to body and mind. In order that any
mode of exercise should be beneficial to persons
of much mental activity, it should have some
provision for entertaining the mind ; for if this is
allowed to be busy as ever, it is not easy to see
how it can be profited by the physical exercise,
and yet nothing is more common than this sort
of practical absurdity. Who does not sometimes
meet, out upon his solitary, solemn walk, some
thin, pale clergyman, for instance, whose every
step and look show that he is meditating on his
next Sunday's sermon ? And yet the good man
flatters himself that he is engaged in a very salutary performance, and goes to his grave, perhaps, without discovering his fatal mistake.
Once observing a friend of mine, who spent a

great part of the day in his counting-room, looking very poorly, I made some inquiries respecting his habits of exercise. He replied, " I am in the saddle one or two hours every day, but the ride does me no good, because it does not divert my mind from its customary thoughts. I know what I need, and I must have it." Accordingly, he went to Scotland, his native land, took a place in the country, engaged in field-sports every day, and within a couple of years found his health completely reëstablished. Let your exercise then be taken in cheerful company, or coupled with a useful errand, or made incidental to some interesting employment. You will soon discern the difference between a walk in the country with no other object than locomotion, and one which contributes something to your collection of plants or minerals, or to the contents of your portfolio.

Among other agencies that affect the health of the mind, none exerts a wider influence, probably, than the diet. Such is not the common sentiment, however, and many a man who admits that improper food may produce bodily illness, will deny, practically, at least, that it can impair the vigor of the mind. The fact that the digestive organs indicate considerable variety in the kind of food suitable for nutrition, taken in connection with the power possessed

by the constitution of adapting itself to a variety of circumstances, have led to a remarkable
laxity of notions on this subject. In the more
popular views, we recognize the influence of
appetite or fashion, rather than that of philosophy or mature experience. I have already alluded to the common proneness of men to suppose that an organic law has not been infringed,
merely because the event has not been signal-
ized by some sudden and striking phenomenon.
Hence it is, chiefly, that no system of diet, however rigid and exclusive, has been without its
votaries, and no article of food or drink so pernicious that it has failed to be extensively used.
Still the great principles of physiology endure,
and if we believe in them, we must be satisfied
that what a man habitually eats and drinks will,
sooner or later, for good or for ill, affect the
health both of body and mind.

Creatures of circumstance as we are, living in
a highly artificial condition, endowed with a
constitution which shows in its inmost germs
the marks of this condition, it is impossible to
lay down any exclusive rules on the subject.
The most we can do will be to bring forward
some general considerations that may help us,
with a little discretion, to a safe practical result.
If it were a question respecting the diet of an
Esquimaux, or an African negro, we should

have no difficulty in deciding it, because it would be fair to conclude that the food most easily accessible, if not the only kind within his reach, is best adapted to his constitution. But when we entertain the same question with respect to a class of people surrounded by every variety of food and climate, with tastes, habits, and faculties infinitely diversified by education, and by those organic influences which are included in the term *domestication*, we are sensible of encountering a problem that scarcely admits of a thorough solution, — a problem that becomes still more difficult when we add to the circumstances here mentioned that of excessive mental application, conjoined with much physical inactivity. Everybody knows that no rule of diet can be of universal application under all this variety of circumstance. The colder the weather, for instance, other things being equal, the greater will be the amount of stimulating food required to maintain the animal heat and repair the waste of organic material. The hardy lumberman in an Eastern forest, under the drafts made upon his forces by extreme cold and immense labor, will consume prodigious quantities of salt pork, and fat of every kind, and evidently thrive upon it. But such a fact does not show what would be the most suitable diet for others, any more than would the dietary of those sanguine reformers who would have us fulfil our duties to the world with only such re-freshment to the inner man as it can derive from sawdust and cold water. After making all due allowance for diversity of circumstances, we venture to lay down the general rule, that the diet most conducive to bodily health and vigor, where the bodily powers chiefly are exercised, will be found, on the whole, most conducive to the mental health and vigor of those who are chiefly engaged in mental employments, though the former, no doubt, may require more. If this proposition excites any surprise, it must be owing to the popular impression that hard-working men require much larger quantities of animal food than they whose employments are of a sedentary character. This popular im-pression, though received with all the authority of an axiom, is founded less upon a careful in-duction of facts than upon a figure of speech. Strong men, it is said, must need have strong food. In this country, a large portion of the diet of the laboring classes consists of animal substances. In Europe, on the contrary, most of the laboring people seldom taste of animal food. It becomes then simply a question of fact, which of the two accomplishes most, and enjoys the greatest measure of health. I am not aware that any inquiries have been made expressly for the purpose of answering this question, but the few observations that have met my notice are very decisive so far as they go. The late Henry Coleman, in one of his agricultural tours, observed that the Scotch farm laborers live almost entirely on oatmeal, scarcely seeing meat through the whole season. He was satisfied that no men do more work, or show better health. This story would be quite incredible to an American laborer, who would sooner believe all the legends of the Talmud than that a good day's work could be performed without an unlimited supply of beef and pork. A hale Scotch gardener, between fifty and sixty years old, told me that, until he came to this country, which was at the age of twenty-seven, he had seldom tasted animal food, yet he was always well, and did as much work as he since had on a very different diet. It is said that in the California mines no class of persons better endure hardships, or accomplish greater results, than the Chinese, and they live chiefly on vegetable food. It is also pertinent to the point to mention, that the standard of health is much lower among our people, probably, than among those just named. They are subject to temporary illnesses causing an inability to work, to a degree that could hardly be expected in a people so early inured to exposure and toil, and so

6

little acquainted with enervating indulgences. The nature of these ailments point, for the most part, to a digestive origin, and may be fairly attributed to errors of diet, of which the principal is a larger amount of animal substances than the organs can easily elaborate. Without laying down any theory of diet, we seem to be warranted in concluding that all classes of persons among us consume a much larger amount of animal food than is really conducive to their bodily health and vigor. I say all classes, because if the proposition be true of those whose labors induce the greatest waste of material, it certainly must be, for a stronger reason, of those whose occupations are light and sedentary. I have been thus particular on this point, because it furnishes us with the surest clew to the solution of the question in hand.

It is a doctrine not calculated to challenge universal assent, that a man of stout limbs and stalwart frame, delving with all his might six days out of seven, needs no more animal food than the attenuated philosopher whose labors are all of the head. Unquestionably one will require more nutriment than the other; but it is only to beg the question to say, that the amount of nutriment is proportioned to the amount of animal food. In the popular notions on this subject, and in some of higher pretensions, we

perceive this fallacy, which seems to have
sprung from some fanciful connection between
muscular strength and animal substance. There
is no necessity for believing that the supply required by the waste of material which physical
exercise produces, cannot be as effectually furnished by vegetable as by animal substances.
We certainly do not believe it in regard to the
domestic animals that share the labors of man,
and which are capable of an amount of physical
power and endurance far beyond the reach of
any carnivorous creature. If this is the law in
regard to the inferior animals, what reason is
there for supposing that it is not also the law in
regard to man? From these considerations we
are led again to the general conclusion, that the
same kind of food which is found most conducive to the bodily health and vigor will also be
found, other things equal, most conducive to
the health and vigor of the mind. I would not
be understood to advocate a strict uniformity of
diet, still less, any sudden changes of diet not
called for by some special exigency. Long-es-
tablished habits are a second nature, and cannot
be disregarded with impunity. I have reference
to the constitution in its normal state, before it
has been weakened and perverted by wrong
habits and hereditary infirmity.

In a dietetic point of view, the drink is no less

important than the solid food. And we are impelled to the same conclusion which seems to
be the true one in regard to food generally, viz.
that whatever best promotes the health of the
body will also best promote the health and vigor
of the mind. It has not yet been satisfactorily
proved that alcoholic drinks are a salutary bev-
erage to persons enjoying a tolerable measure of
health, and working within an easy round of
employment. Still, it is a fair question, whether, under the influences of civilization — which
bears the same relation to man that domestication does to the inferior animals — the human
constitution has not become so changed from
the normal condition as to require a diet somewhat different from that most suitable in its
original state. The ox and the horse in their
native abodes thrived on grass and shrubs, but
this would be indifferent provender to the horse
and ox of our times. The fruits of the field and
the crystal stream may have been amply sufficient for man in his state of primeval innocence, but does he not, under the wear and tear
of civilized life, require a diet more substantial
and stimulating, like the creatures just mentioned ? Are not tea, coffee, wine, and spirits
necessary, in some degree, to maintain the
bodily and mental powers in their most vigorous
condition amid the exhausting influences — the

duties, the pleasures, the joys and the sorrows,
the toil and the conflict — of artificial life?
The principle involved in the question seems to
be clear enough. If the powers are habitually
urged beyond an easy activity, or the stamina of
the constitution have become enfeebled by hereditary defects, those articles may be salutary
just as medicine is salutary when actual disease
is present. It is but an illustration of the great
law that pervades all nature, that one abuse
necessarily leads to another. The practical application of the principle is not so clear. The
precise amount of mental exhaustion, of enervating habits, of constitutional infirmity, that
may seem to require a supply of artificial stimulus, is not very easily settled. With every
disposition to judge correctly, the rigid moralist
would probably place it too low, while the *bon
vivant* would err in the opposite direction; and
the latter error would, unquestionably, be the
more common. The history of literary men
shows very strongly that the exercise of the
highest powers of the mind, through a long life,
does not necessarily require much if any alcoholic stimulus. In fact, they who have labored
hardest and longest were singularly abstemious.
Newton, Locke, Gibbon, Burke, Scott, were
among the most temperate of men; and yet, if
the amount of intellectual labor is to decide the

amount of indulgence, certainly none could have
claimed more than these celebrated men. If intellectual labor ever exhausts the nervous energies to such a degree, that stimulating drinks
are required to sustain them at the working
point, it must be supposed to have done it in
their cases. True, they were not teetotalers,
and it never can be proved that they would have
done equally well without the little which they
took. They were satisfied, it may be said, with
that moderate indulgence which kept the nervous system in its best possible tone without
exceeding the limits of a healthy stimulation.
There is much reason to believe, however, that
the habits of those men arose, less from any instinctive cravings, than from the conventional
usages of the sphere in which they moved, and
consequently might have been abandoned entirely
without any detriment to their mental health.
and energy. Cases there have been, no doubt,
where great intellectual efforts were rendered
possible only by the liberal use of stimulating
drinks. Pitt, during the latter years of his life,
if not before, never encountered the labor and
excitement of a parliamentary debate without
enormous libations of port wine. Two or three
bottles of a night, accompanied by a beefsteak,
was the usual allowance, and undoubtedly he
would have been powerless without it. It would

have required a stouter constitution than Pitt's
to stand the wear and tear of such duties and
such habits beyond the age of forty-five. Instead of holding up his case as an example to
be followed, or as a proof that indulgence to
any degree is favorable to mental energy, I
would rather have it regarded as an example of
injudicious training, premature effort, and pernicious habits, to be most carefully pondered
and avoided. A better example, both in morals
and hygiene, was exhibited by his illustrious
compeer, Burke, who met the same kind of demand upon his energies by no stronger stimulus
than hot water.

If it be true that men like Burke, and others
moving in a similar sphere, really need no alcoholic stimulus, should we not hesitate to recom-
mend it to that numerous class whose business
requires the intense application of their minds,
many hours in the day, under circumstances not
very favorable to their physical health? It is
not an uncommon opinion, that many of these
persons would break down without the aid
afforded by such stimulus, and I rather believe
it has some foundation in fact. When men
habitually overtask their brains, and accompany
their imprudence by a disregard of many other
rules of health, they may, not improbably, prolong a precarious existence by resorting to such

means. Other persons, too, more prudent in
managing their mental resources, who feel the
depressing effects of civic life, and find relief
from the use of stimulating drinks, are liable to
adopt the idea that they may be equally salutary
as a prophylactic after the casual ailment has
passed away. Such means of preserving the
health is far more agreeable to most men, than
air, exercise, and recreation, which require time,
opportunity, and self-denial; and here is the
source of much of the self-deception which pervades this subject. To the young who are sincerely seeking the right course in regard to the
use of stimulating drinks, I do not hesitate to
say, as the result to which the most careful and
candid observers have arrived, You may safely
resolve to abstain entirely, until advised to the
contrary by a competent physician.

Knowing what we do of the organic laws, we
are obliged to believe that the habitual use of
spirituous liquors must necessarily impair the
health of the brain, and thus disturb its functions. That it engenders disease of the stomach, liver, and some other organs, is a fact well
established by anatomical researches; but its
immediate effect on the brain, as indicated by
the mental manifestations, is too obvious to require any research at all. Now, this frequent
stimulation of the cerebral organism is unnatu-

ral, and, like all unnatural actions in the animal
economy, must be detrimental to its energy and
vigor. The general law is, that any organ habitually stimulated beyond a certain point thereby loses its natural energy, and sooner or later
becomes the seat of disease. In no other organ
is the operation of this law more speedy or severe. To say that a brain which has been much
stimulated by strong drink will continue to perform its functions with undiminished power, is
to affirm what is not sustained by actual experience, or the laws of the animal economy.

These remarks, it must be understood, apply
to those only who are supposed to be sound
and healthy. To those, on the contrary, whose
vital energies have been impaired by disease or
exhausting labors, the regulated use of alcoholic stimulants may be required to supply the
waste of the nervous forces incident to intellectual labors. In this abnormal condition of
the system, the unassisted efforts of nature
would fail to maintain the mind at its working
point, or even to restore the physical vigor. No
medical man, not wedded to a theory, will deny
the correctness of this statement, for that experience must have been very peculiar which has
not furnished abundant illustrations. Indeed,
we might, with as little regard for the results
of experience, deny that bark can stop the par-

oxyms of intermittent fever, or that opium can produce sleep and nervous tranquillity.

There is a form of mental disorder produced by intemperate habits, and now become deplorably common, which may be properly noticed in this connection. I refer to that insatiable propensity to drink which impels the person to indulge, in spite of the strongest possible inducements to refrain, as if the will were powerless, and the moral sense somewhat blunted. It differs from the ordinary fondness for drink — in which, no doubt, it generally originates — in being beyond the control of any conceivable moral consideration, and connected, probably, with some pathological condition of the brain. It is manifested under two general forms. In one, the person proceeds from one excess to another and a greater, until a maniacal condition of the brain is produced, when he becomes unconscious of his acts, and, often, disposed to violence. In the other, he retires to some secluded place, and there, quietly and alone, rapidly imbibes large quantities of liquor, until the stomach refuses to receive any more. He then remains for a time in a stupid, listless state, which is succeeded by the natural condition, and this, after an interval more or less brief, by a repetition of the same scenes. In both cases, the individual seems to have no more moral free-

dom than the true maniac has while committing
his extravagances. He is entirely under the dominion of an organic impulse by which he is
led automatically, and sometimes unconsciously.
In the early stages of the paroxysm, he may appear to be aware of what he is about, and fancy
that he is only indulging within reasonable limits.
He feels quite secure, and every remonstrance is
indignantly answered in a tone of injured innocence. Or he may admit, to the fullest extent,
the enormity of his sin and his peril, while he
deplores his utter inability to resist the appetite
that rages within him. One whose case is related by Macnish, thus replied to the remonstrances
of his friend: " Your remarks are just; they are,
indeed, too true ; but I can no longer resist temptation. If a bottle of brandy stood at one hand,
and the pit of hell yawned at the other, and I
were convinced that I would be pushed in as
sure as I took one glass, I could not refrain.
You are very kind: I ought to be very grate-
ful for so many kind, good friends, but you may
spare yourselves the trouble of trying to reform
me ; the thing is out of the question."* And thus
it is, that advice, admonition, and reproach are
all equally lost upon this class of persons, and
the end is the same in nearly all, — they lose all
rational control over their conduct, abandon their

---

* *Anatomy of Drunkenness*, Chap. xiv.

employments, desert or abuse their families, and
though they commit no act of violence, they, at
least, destroy the peace and threaten the safety
of those around them.

In some cases the propensity seems to be excited by some moral cause which severely tries
the mental energies, such as unusual responsibility, excessive mental application, the person,
generally, not being an habitual drinker.   Indeed, in the severest case that ever came to my
knowledge, the person had previously scarcely
known the taste of intoxicating drinks; and in
the intervals between his paroxysms, nothing
could induce him to indulge in the slightest
degree.

An evil so common as this has become, and
so sad in its consequences to all concerned, is
justly regarded with the deepest interest, by
every friend of man; and during the last forty
or fifty years, few questions have agitated the
community more than those which relate to its
prevention or cure.   Magistrates, legislators, moralists, philanthropists, have tasked their ingenuity in devising modes of relief; and in the various
attempts to accomplish so desirable and so difficult an end, every conceivable motive by which
men are usually actuated, has been addressed,
with what success I need not say.

With the means of prevention, I have here no

concern, and in regard to the means of cure, which do come within my province, I fear I can offer nothing very satisfactory. The pathological element in this condition would seem to imply the propriety of medical treatment, but the difficulty here is, that the patient is unwilling or unable to take the first step in the treatment of any disease, — that of removing the cause of the disease. To secure this object, as well as to prevent the mischief liable to arise from the frenzy that often exists, it is necessary sometimes to subject the patient to restraint and confinement; and inasmuch as his domestic arrangements might render this impossible in his own home or any private family, hospitals for the insane have been resorted to, of late years, for this purpose. They furnish the rest and effect the abstinence that are required, and if the person can be kept sufficiently long, the best results may sometimes be obtained. There are objections, however, to this measure, some real and others fanciful, which have led to other projects. Some of these persons are very unfit associates with the insane, and thus the legitimate purpose of these institutions is, to that extent, frustrated. On the other hand, some of them feel, or profess to feel, outraged by being compelled to witness scenes which shock their sensibilities and render them constantly uncomfortable and unhappy;

though, as a matter of fact, such are the means
of classification in most of our hospitals for the
insane, that they need see but little, if any, more
of insanity, or, at least, of its prominent features,
than they would in the world at large.

The last project taken into favor, for dealing
with the evil in question, is that of establishments expressly designed for the reception and
treatment of inebriates. What their success
may be is a matter of speculation, as no one
of much consequence has yet been opened.
They certainly are exempt from the objections
just mentioned as lying against hospitals for the
insane, but it can hardly be supposed that they
would be entirely exempt from social annoyances
more disagreeable even than any that can arise
from association with the insane. But this is
not all. In their special work, they must labor
under the same difficulty as hospitals for the insane, — the difficulty of retaining their cases sufficiently long to make a permanent impression.
Even the most of those who would consent to the
step, while suffering under the peculiar wretchedness incident to their propensity, have no idea
of prolonging their seclusion after the immediate
effects of indulgence have disappeared. The
restoration of the bodily condition to something
like its customary strength and firmness, with
all the pleasing sensations which follow such a

change, excite no distrust of their power to resist temptation. On the contrary, they are always hopeful, confident, sanguine, and impatient of delay. They say they feel perfectly well, have not the slightest desire for drink, and, therefore, that farther seclusion would be, not only unnecessary, but prejudicial to their mental and bodily health. The amazing confidence such persons invariably express in their future security, is one of the curious traits of this condition. A great many have come under my observation, but I never knew one — not even of those who had repeatedly fallen, and had most deplored their infirmity — to express any apprehension of falling again. On the contrary, from the moment when they begin to resume their proper consciousness until they leave the hospital, the burden of their story is, that they are safe forever after; that not the slightest danger exists of their again disregarding the terrible lessons of experience. Instead of returning into the world with fear and trembling, as one would naturally expect to see them, and seizing upon any excuse for postponing the day of trial, they go out eager and jubilant, as if bound on a festive excursion.

Thus beguiled by a morbid confidence in themselves, they determine to reassume their liberty, in spite of entreaty and argument, and the institution has no power to prevent it. Neither a

hospital for the insane nor an asylum for inebriates can hold persons in confinement against
their consent, for any other cause than insanity;
and though our account of this class of persons
does not indicate in them a very healthy condition of mind, yet, inasmuch as they are apparently rational after the first day or two, both in
conduct and conversation, they cannot be called
insane, in the ordinary acceptation of the term.
While in the paroxysm, or suffering under its
immediate effects, they may, very properly, be
called insane, and so long they may, unquestionably, be deprived of their liberty, for the purposes
of custody or cure. But when this condition
shall have passed away, forcible detention in any
institution, whatever it may be called, would be
clearly a violation of constitutional rights, and
would not be sanctioned by the legal tribunals.

A notion prevails, I am aware, that the ine-
briate asylum is to be unprovided with bolts,
bars, and guards, and no means of detention allowed more forcible than the offices of kindness,
good-will, and love. Respecting this notion it
need only be said that it indicates but a school-
boy's knowledge of human nature, and a still
deeper ignorance of that special phasis of it
which results from long-continued, irresistible
inebriety.

The spectacle is a sad one, and no reliable

promise of relief appears in any quarter whatever, but we may be allowed to hope that in the infinite resources of Providence, means will be afforded for restraining, if not abolishing, this tremendous evil.

There remains to be considered one more physical agency closely connected with the health of the brain, — sleep. A periodical renewal of the nervous energies as often as once a day is an institution of nature, none the less necessary to the well-being of the animal economy, because in some degree under the control of the will. To disregard its requirements with impunity is no more possible than it is to violate any other organic law with impunity; and no man need flatter himself that he may systematically intrench upon the hours usually devoted to rest, and still retain the freshness and elasticity of his faculties. With the same kindliness that marks all the arrangements of the animal economy, this condition is attended with many pleasing sensations and salutary effects, gently alluring us to seek the renovation which it offers. " While I am asleep," says the immortal Sancho Panza, " I have neither fear nor hope, neither trouble nor glory ; and blessings on him who invented sleep, — the mantle that covers all human thoughts ; the food that appeases hunger ; the drink that quenches thirst ; the fire

7

that warms cold; the cold that moderates heat;
and, lastly, the general coin that purchases all
things; — the balance and weight that make the
shepherd equal to the king, and the simple to
the wise." The ill effects of insufficient sleep
may be witnessed on some of the principal organic functions, but it is the brain and nervous
system that suffer chiefly and in the first instance. The consequences of a very protracted
vigil are too well known to be mistaken, but
many a person is suffering, unconscious of the
cause, from the habit of irregular and insufficient
sleep. One of its most common effects is a degree of nervous irritability and peevishness which
even the happiest self-discipline can scarcely
control. That buoyancy of the feelings, that
cheerful, hopeful, trusting temper that springs far
more from organic conditions than from mature
and definite convictions, give way to a spirit
of dissatisfaction and dejection; while the even
demeanor, the measured activity, are replaced,
either by a lassitude that renders any exertion
painful, or an impatience and restlessness not
very conducive to happiness. Upon the intellectual powers the mischief is still more serious.
They not only lose that healthy activity which
combines and regulates their movements in the
happiest manner, but they are no longer capable
of efforts once perfectly easy. The conceptions

cease to be clear and well-defined, the power of endurance is weakened, inward perceptions are confounded with outward impressions, and illusory images obtrude themselves unbidden upon the mind. This kind of disturbance may pass, sooner or later, into actual insanity, and many a noble spirit has been utterly prostrated by habitual loss of rest. Southey, whom no amount of literary labor seemed to fatigue, sunk under its disastrous effects; and this it was that caused his hardy intellect, that had successfully encountered adversity and trial, to go down at last in clouds and darkness. After the labors of the day, he was accustomed, very often, to watch, the greater part of the night, by the bed of his first wife, through a protracted illness; and thus, his friend Wordsworth thought, he prepared for the calamity that finally overtook him. * Even the gigantic intellect of Newton reeled under the shock of a similar trial. In September, 1693, he conceived that Locke and other friends were endeavoring to embroil him with the government, and that the former was writing books that struck at the root of morality. On the 5th of October following, he wrote a letter to Locke, in which he says: " The last winter, by sleeping too often by my fire, I got an ill habit of sleeping; and a

* *Scenery and Poetry of the English Lakes*, by C. Mackay.

distemper, which, this summer, has been epidemical, put me farther out of order; so that
when I wrote to you, I had not slept an hour a
night for a fortnight together, and, for five days
together, not a wink. I remember I wrote to
you, but what I said of your book I remember
not." *

Where a predisposition to insanity exists,
nothing proves to be a more potent exciting
cause than the loss of sleep. Persons thus unfortunately constituted must beware how they
allow their duties or pleasures to interfere with
this restorative process which is indispensable
even to their present safety. The records of
our asylums show that in a large proportion of
cases the disease was attributable chiefly to this
cause, which a little more prudence would
have prevented.

The amount of sleep necessary to good health
must vary, like food and exercise, in different
individuals, according to their duties, temper-
aments, and habits. Some are capable of accomplishing much with very little sleep, and apparently suffer no harm. Pichegru, the French
revolutionary general, went through a year's
campaign, sleeping but one hour in the twenty-
four, and still enjoying good health. After making all suitable allowances, we are inclined to

* Brewster's *Life of Newton*, II. 240.

believe that from six to eight hours of sleep are necessary to the highest condition of bodily and mental health. Sleep, however, unlike food and exercise, cannot always be regulated by the will. From one cause or another, every person is unable at times to obtain the amount of sleep he requires. In vain we court the favors of the drowsy god. The more anxiously they are sought, the less readily do they come at our bidding, and much of the night is spent in solitary vigils that recruit neither body nor mind. Sooner or later, the consequences of this condition, if it continue long, become visible in some form of impaired mental vigor.

The practical lesson taught by such facts is, that we should avoid all those habits that are manifestly unfavorable to sound sleep, and practise every appropriate art for obtaining it. The empire of prejudice, habit, fashion, and social arrangement, is too strong, I fear, to be weakened by the counsels of the physician, but this would scarcely excuse us in passing over in silence a matter of so much importance. With many persons devoted to intellectual pursuits, the night is the favorite period of study and composition. They have forced themselves to believe that they cannot possibly think or write with fluency or fervor at any other period; as if the noblest exercise of the intellect could be pursued only under circumstances incompatible with its health and vigor. The idea that one can use his mind only at a certain time of day is a whim unworthy of a rational being, and indicative of the most imperfect self-discipline. Let him who would derive the highest satisfaction from intellectual pursuits learn to be independent of the petty accidents of time and place, and be assured that, until he has accomplished this lesson, he is not master of himself. They who pursue this habit of night-study, pass directly from their desks to their beds. In some few happily constituted individuals, the transition from the highest mental activity to a state of absolute repose is the work of a moment, but with most persons it is a long and difficult process. The tension of the nervous fibres will not relax immediately, the images that have been thronging the brain refuse to depart, and no effort of will can induce that unconsciousness which comes unbidden, if it come at all. Boerhaave relates that having once indulged from morning till night in intense thought, he did not close his eyes for six weeks, during all which time he was indifferent to everything. This practice must be abandoned if we would insure sound sleep. It is a good general rule to spend the last hour or two before retiring to rest in some form of recreation, or the lightest kind of mental exercise; and it is also another good rule to retire early.

Looking at the affluent classes generally, it is obvious that the social customs of the time are quite incompatible with those habits of rest which are essential to mental vigor. The late hours which most forms of evening amusement, or other social gathering, require, sadly en-croach upon the time that should be allotted to rest, and the calls of business do not always al-low the deficiency to be met by abstracting ever so little from the golden hours of morning. Besides this, in the young and inexperienced, the scenes of the evening are not readily effaced from the mind, but pass and repass before it, in all the vividness of reality, long after the eyes have been closed, and the hovering slumbers in-vited to descend. The brain is in no condition for sleep. The circulation is accelerated, and the nervous system excited; sleep, when it comes, if it come at all, is fitful, and disturbed by dreams; the person rises but little refreshed by this abortive attempt at repose, and the du-ties of the day are pursued under a sense of languor, if not positive weariness. True, a few nights of uninterrupted repose may repair ap-parently the evil of a single indulgence, and were it limited to a single indulgence once or twice a year, the effect might be scarcely appreciable. But where such amusements are pursued very frequently, perhaps night after night for a whole season together, they make a very considerable addition to the amount of nervous depreciation inseparable from the habits of a highly civilized life. This cause alone is accountable for much of the ill-health that prevails among the easier classes, and always must, so long as the law of our nature requires regular and sufficient sleep.

The efficiency of the mind as a working power, will be affected, in a very great degree, by the stint of mental exercise to which it is subjected. A fruitful source of mental impairment is the prevalent mistake of supposing that the brain possesses a power of exertion and endurance unlimited by any other law than our own free will and pleasure. Here we disregard those laws of health which we respect in the exercise of other organs; and many a man who would shrink from the folly of habitually cramming his stomach with food, or of changing his dress incautiously, will work his brain every day beyond the point of fatigue; not even manifesting the prudence with which he would use the most common machine subject to the wear and tear resulting from friction and decay. In every department of mental exertion, we witness this serious mistake. The lawyer, the doctor, the minister, the scholar, the merchant, the mechanic, all apparently act on the presumption that their brains are made of iron, which no conceivable amount of use can weaken or derange. In many of them, the brain is kept in a state of incessant activity, often of the most wearing description, during the greater part of the day. As a consequence of such habits, it is not strange that every description of mental infirmity should have increased among us of late, to an extent that has no parallel in former times. In the prime of life, in the midst of usefulness, men rapidly break down, and, after hovering around their customary haunts for a brief period, disappear forever. By insanity, paralysis, and other organic lesions, brains are now "used up," in the popular phrase, with a frequency that is full of instruction, if we would but heed it. Paralytic affections, which once were comparatively rare, and attributable in great part to hereditary predisposition or sensual indulgences, now occur in multitudes who seemed to be enjoying good health and had always been regular and temperate in all their ways. Indeed, were we to indicate that feature in the medical constitution of our times, which distinguishes it from all others, it would be our large proportion of cerebral affections.

It can scarcely be doubted, however, that a
certain amount of mental activity is necessary
in order to obtain the highest degree of mental
health. Although excessive exercise of the
mind, as we have seen, is calculated to impair
its efficiency, yet it is no less certain that the
worst results sometimes follow excessive inactivity and listlessness. It might be supposed,
perhaps, that a person whose thoughts never extend beyond a very limited range, would never
suffer from mental disorder ; and the remarkable
exemption of savage tribes from diseases of the
mind would seem to confirm this idea. But all
the analogies of physiology show that an organ
which is little used gradually loses its efficiency,
and assumes that molecular arrangement which
invites the approach of disease; and if the savage is more exempt than the sage from mental
infirmities, as he probably is, the fact is to be
attributed to his greater exemption from all the
deteriorating influences of civilization, whereby
his brain, as well as all the other organs, enjoys
the largest possible measure of health. In persons of a dull, narrow understanding, and predisposed also in any degree to mental affections,
the lack of sufficient mental exercise may constitute the single agency that is required to convert this tendency into overt disease, by reason
of the same organic law whereby the same dis-

aster is made to follow excessive use of the
mind. In every old community are people of
this description, who feel no interest in anything
beyond their own little circle, — whose wishes
and sympathies and aspirations never extend
beyond the confines of their farm or workshop.
They plod on from day to day in the old beaten
track, while the clamor of the world around
them falls on their ear, exciting as little emotion as the roar of the angry ocean in the sleeping mariner. The discoveries of art and science
excite no curiosity ; the achievements of philanthropy touch no responsive chord; and the great
events of their time — a decisive battle, or the
dismemberment of an empire — are regarded as
no concern of theirs. This kind of indifference
is not the result of philosophy, nor of proper attention to their own affairs. It is an apathy depending on defective cerebral energy, liable, on
the occurrence of the first adverse incident, to
be converted into active disease. Every hospital in the land abounds with representatives of
this class, especially from the older parts of the
country, where things have become somewhat
fixed, and life flows on with the least possible
amount of distraction. In settling the general
question of the utility of lectures and gatherings
and public amusements, their hygienic effect in
quickening the torpid energies of such persons

ought not to be overlooked. They might serve to kindle a little emotion, or excite a little intellectual effort, and thus prevent the current of their mental life from becoming utterly stagnant.

At what age precisely the mind enjoys its highest vigor, is capable of the greatest efforts and the greatest endurance, is a question that cannot be very definitely answered, and yet it would seem as if some standard should be fixed upon whereby to graduate the degree of mental application at the different periods of life. Examples are not rare of elderly scholars, especially in Germany, who habitually devoted twelve or fourteen hours a day to hard study. A distinguished American jurist was accustomed, for several years immediately preceding his death, which occurred after the age of seventy, to spend fourteen hours a day in writing an historical work, and in other literary employment. No class of men, probably, perform so great an amount of intellectual labor as English and American judges, sitting in court, as they do, a large part of their time, six or eight hours a day, with their minds constantly on the stretch, amid the disadvantages of badly warmed, badly ventilated apartments; and thence retiring to their chambers, perhaps, to investigate a question of law, or prepare a judg-

ment. The most of these men are past the me-
ridian of life. It is not quite certain, however,
that such labors do not make serious drafts on
the constitution. Instances that seem to show
a different result are, probably, exceptions to the
general rule.

There is much reason to believe that the development of mental power proceeds, by equal
steps, with that of the body, — that it is precisely at that period when the physical powers
are most mature, that the mind is capable of the
most close and successful application. No one
would think of looking for this period after the
age of forty-five ; and as little should we look
for it, notwithstanding the achievements of
some youthful Hercules, on the earlier side of
twenty. Power of physical endurance, of meeting that wear and tear of the vital forces that
results from continuous and protracted activity,
proceeds from a certain maturity of the bodily
organization, and that strength which only habitual trial can generate. Before the age of
twenty, this kind of maturity and strength is seldom witnessed ; and experiments made on a
large scale, as in war and colonization, furnish
abundant proof of this fact. During the last
years of the first French Empire, when the con-
scriptions were frequently anticipated in order
to supply the frightful waste of life produced by

its sanguinary wars, Napoleon often complained that the young conscripts they sent him were fit only to encumber the hospitals and road-sides. During the period, then, varying not far from thirty on the one side, and forty-five on the other, the body enjoys its maximum of vigor and power of endurance; and it is during this period that the history of studious men leads us to believe that the mind displays corresponding attributes. Of course this is meant for a general statement only, to which there are numerous exceptions. The history of literary and scientific men furnishes many an illustrious example of intellectual power undimmed and undiminished by the influences of old age. Bacon, Milton, Burke, Cuvier, exhibited, to the very last the same ability which distinguished their earlier years. It may be doubted, however, whether this kind of exemption from the effects of age is not chiefly confined to men of extraordinary endowments. They are too few, perhaps, to furnish the ground of a fair comparison; but, certainly, it is difficult to point out a single instance of such a man exhibiting, with increase of years, indications of mental deterioration, while they are common enough among the inferior grades of intellect.

How much a man may use his brain without endangering its health, is a question that admits of no definite answer, because it depends very much on the original stamina of the individual, and the intensity of his application. While it is easy, oftentimes, to see that this or that person is overtasking his powers, it is impossible to lay down any general rule on the subject that would not require too much of some and too little of others. In youth and early manhood, especially if the constitution is deficient in vigor, there would be danger from a degree of application, that might be safe enough at a later period, when the brain has become hardened by age and regular labor. So, too, habits of active physical exercise will enable a man to accomplish an amount of intellectual labor that would utterly break down one of sedentary habits. After making all due allowance for these differences, I think we may say, that few can exceed six hours a day of close mental application, without seriously endangering the health of the brain, while for most persons a not unreasonable degree of prudence would prescribe a much shorter period. It would not be easy to adduce many instances of persons who, for some length of time, had devoted more than six hours a day to pursuits requiring the exercise of the higher intellectual faculties, without impairing their powers, and failing to accomplish any results corresponding to the magnitude of their efforts.

We hear, indeed, of persons studying ten or
twelve hours in the day, but, with an occasional
exception, it may well be doubted whether
more would not be actually accomplished
within shorter limits. In most persons, long before this period is finished, the process of thinking goes on heavily, the mind loses its power of
original conception; and the result of its labors,
while in this jaded condition, lacking the vigor
and brilliancy of a fresh effort, is said to smell
of the lamp.

Men who have been long accustomed to write
books, and experience a certain pleasure in the
exercise, unite in declaring that five or six hours
a day in the labor of composition, year in and
year out, cannot be profitably exceeded. Sir
Walter Scott, than whom few literary men
have accomplished a greater amount of intellectual labor, by reason of a naturally strong constitution, good habits of exercise and recreation,
and a cheerful tone of mind, emphatically de-
clared that six hours a day was the utmost limit
of his taskwork; and the correctness of his
statement was painfully verified in the latter
part of his career, when the desire of retrieving
his fortunes induced him to exceed this stint.
The melancholy result is known to every one,
and it forms a chapter in literary history unsurpassed by any other in its deep, tragic interest.

His health soon suffered, and that noble intellect which seemed almost beyond the reach of blight or decay, utterly broke down and passed away. It may be said, perhaps, that Scott was engaged in the most exhausting description of mental exercise, — the composition of works that the world will not soon forget, — and, consequently, was unable to prolong his working hours to a limit quite safe for those whose mental labors consist merely in adding up figures, in counting money, or any other intellectual drudgery. There is something in this, no doubt; but it must be considered that if his work were more arduous, the power of accomplishing it derived from vigorous health, a cheerful temperament, active exercise, and strict temperance, has seldom been equalled. Those civic pursuits which keep the mind on the stretch for six or eight hours a day are accompanied by few of those advantages, and the daily waste of nervous energy is not repaired, as far as it might be, by appropriate habits of living. In our principal towns and cities, the period allotted to business of one kind or another, is from six to ten hours a day. During all this time the mind may not be engaged in the severest kind of exercise — although with many this is actually so — but it is constantly on the alert, and under a pressure of excitement. With a very large proportion of men, life is a constant struggle with circumstances, not confined entirely to hours of business. The objects they have set before them, whether near or remote, are surrounded with difficulties that cannot be overcome without effort nor contemplated without anxiety. Every day is laden with some new experience of hopes deferred or fulfilled, of enterprises that have failed or succeeded, of labor crowned by abundant fruit or followed by barren results. The class in question embraces, not merely those who are aiming at the glittering prizes of life, but the countless multitude who, with humbler views, are still endeavoring, to use the popular phrase, to better their condition. They make no mark upon the world; indeed they are scarcely noticed amid the crowds that throng the great avenues of life, but to each belongs a brain throbbing with every pulse of the swelling tide that leads on to wealth, honor, or distinction. Their number is constantly increased by all the tendencies of the age, but the power to meet this draft upon their mental energies is not increased by judicious training or proper self-discipline. I need not say how imperfectly any stated period of time can indicate the exact amount of mental activity to which such people are subject. Long after the visible close of business, the mind is fixed upon the events of

the day, and moments that are supposed to be
given to repose or recreation are still occupied
by the teeming, toiling brain.

I scarcely need remark how often, among
men whose pursuits are exclusively intellectual,
the limit of daily downright work is extended
far beyond six or eight hours. Especially is this
the case in the legal profession. Between con-
sultations in his office, attendance in court, and
the preparation of cases for trial, the lawyer in
full practice is occupied, the greater part of the
time not given to sleep, in mental exercise of
the severest description. In this respect, the bar
is quite equalled by the bench, whose inexorable
duties require an amount of close and continuous application seldom surpassed in any other
department of professional labor. The clergyman of our times, too, especially if he have
achieved any degree of eminence, scarcely has an
easier lot. To supply the weekly tale of rhetoric
and oratory which modern refinement demands,
there is required a degree of mental activity
which, however easy it may become by habitual
practice, is exhausting even to those most happily endowed. When we add to this the many
extraordinary calls that task his powers, and
which must be promptly and discreetly met, and
bear in mind the pernicious habit of night-work
so common with clergymen, as well as their

notorious neglect of the plainest rules of hygiene, we cannot be surprised that their career is so often brief and painful.

In persons who are thus working beyond their strength, there sometimes comes on a kind of nervous erythism which makes them crave the excitement of work as something necessary to their very existence. Scott, while striving with all the might of his marvellous intellect to dis-charge the claims of his creditors, could no longer confine himself to the customary stint of five or six hours. The immense increase of his task-work only stimulated instead of enfeebling his energies, while he shrunk from rest as if it were a forced and unnatural state. His phy-sician remonstrated in vain. " I tell you what it is, doctor," he replied, " Molly, when she puts the kettle on, may just as well say, ' Kettle, kettle, don't boil.' " In a letter to a friend about this time, he says: " Dr. Abercrombie threatens me with death, if I write so much ; and die, I suppose I must, if I give it up suddenly." A gentleman in this city, justly distinguished both in law and literature, in describing his own case, tells the same story in brief but graphic terms: " I begin to think that I am losing the power of rest and repose, and that, like an over-driven cab-horse, I should drop down if taken out of the thills." Cases like these are not confined to the walks of literature. Many a man immersed in the active pursuits of civic life, finds his faculties strained to a degree of tension apparently inevitable, while the idea of relaxation seems to be equivalent to that of dissolution. Such is one of the fearful penalties that follow the violation of that natural law which ordains that work, when carried beyond a certain point, is no longer a source of health and enjoyment.

There is another kind of cerebral labor in regard to which it is of the utmost importance that the theory and practice of the community should be correct, — I mean that which is imposed upon the young in the process of education, under the name of study. To say that it has always or generally been determined by a careful consideration of the laws of physiology, and a scrupulous regard to the results of experience, would be to utter the broadest possible irony. Unfortunately, the question has been almost universally overshadowed by another and a very different one, in most modern communities, viz. what will satisfy the public, — that public which mistakes the glitter of display for solid acquirement, and measures the skill of the teacher by the rapidity with which the pupil is pushed forward. The radical fault is the same which characterizes our movements in other departments of effort. We grudge the time a sound education necessarily requires, and are impatient to turn the acquisitions of the pupil to some practical account. Discipline and development may be theoretically recognized as legitimate objects of education, but, practically, they are subordinate to that which predominates over all others, viz. the means of distinction which it gives, — the medals, prizes, honors. These are to be obtained, if possible, and obtained quickly. Here, as in everything else, speed is the great test of merit. Lesson is piled upon lesson, the hours of study are increased, and the active, irritable brain of tender youth is habitually forced to the utmost power of effort.

Governed by the mechanical spirit of the age, we have formed the habit of regarding the youthful brain in the light of a machine that may be worked to the utmost limit of its capacity. Recreation and rest are regarded as a loss of valuable time, and the lying idle of capital that should be continually productive. This view of the matter arises from the fallacy, that the growth and development of the mind are in exact relation to the amount of task-work it has accomplished. The history of our country, to go no farther, furnishes little support to such a notion. The distinguished men whose early years were spent in an unceasing attendance upon schools and academies, are far outnumbered by those whose means of instruction consisted in a few months' schooling in the winter, and a diligent pondering of such scraps of literature as might be picked out of the basket of the itinerant pedler. If I am told that such men achieve their greatness in spite of the deficiencies of education, and that the benefit of the forcing system is better exhibited in the elevation of an inferior order of minds, I would still reply that the position, even thus modified, finds no stronger support. If we look into the walks of commerce, agriculture, or manufactures, and learn the history of those who, without being great, hold a marked position in society, I think the result of the inquiry will strengthen the view we have taken. Of course, the importance of systematic education cannot be questioned, but it must be borne in mind that the efficiency of education is indicated more by the power and endurance which it imparts than by the amount of its immediate visible effects. Undoubtedly, the tree may be judged by its fruits ; but let us not confound with the ripe and full-grown fruits that crown the harvest, the ephemeral blossoms that excite the admiration of the beholder, and forthwith perish, leaving not a trace behind.

The amount of daily task-work that may be safely required of the young, in the process of

education, may be ascertained with some approach to correctness, by adopting as a standard
of comparison that which is regarded as the
most suitable for the adult mind. Of course, it
should vary somewhat with differences of natural endowment and vigor, but it can scarcely
be questioned that it cannot safely exceed the
limit of greatest performance assigned to the
full-grown intellect.

It may be objected to this conclusion, perhaps, that the exercises of school require no
such strain upon the mind as the effort of composition, especially as the former are chiefly a
matter of memory, and not original creation.
There may be something in this, but not
enough surely to forbid the inference we have
drawn. These lessons of the child are not
merely to be committed to memory and repeated, but they are to be understood, if possible, and this implies the exercise of the higher
faculties of the mind. In the study of languages, for instance, the meaning of words, the
relation of one word to another, the force of
expressions, frequently cannot be ascertained
without reference to cognate words and expressions; and amid a multiplicity of suggestions, some effort of sagacity is required in
order rightly to choose between them. In the
study of mathematics, too, those truths which

seem so obvious when once they are worked out, cannot be mastered without a concentration and continuity of attention, which imply effort and fatigue. In mental science, also, if the performance of the pupil is to be anything better than a parrot-like repetition of what is contained in the book, there must be an effort of abstraction and introspection which, to a young mind totally unaccustomed to such an exercise, is no easy work. Besides, in the two cases supposed, it is to be considered that the writer has the advantage of familiar practice, takes easily to his work, and the toil is lightened and cheered by the hope of substantial reward. Unless, therefore, we greatly misapprehend the nature of the connection between mental activity and the organic condition of the brain, we have a right to conclude, that the youthful powers may be not less severely tried by five or six hours' attention to the above-named studies, than the adult mind by the practice of writing for the same period. But this is not all. The young and the adult brains possess very unequal capacities of application and endurance. It is the law of the animal economy that the various organs do not arrive at their full maturity of vigor and power, until some time after the adult age has fairly commenced. To suppose the youthful brain to be capable of an amount of

task-work which is considered an ample allowance to an adult brain, is simply absurd, and
the attempt to carry this folly into effect must
necessarily be dangerous to the health and efficiency of this organ.

Now let us look at the particular facts in the
case, and see what amount of labor is habitually imposed upon the young, in the shape of
school-exercises ; how much time must be spent
upon them by the mass of the pupils in order to
obtain a respectable standing in the school; and
what is the effect of all this effort on the mental
health.

Six hours a day, for the most part, is the
allotted school-time in this part of the country.   Occasionally we find it five, and as often,
probably, seven.   The rooms, with some rare
exceptions, are badly warmed and badly ventilated, the thermometer ranging, in winter, from
55 to 60, and the air contaminated by the respiration of one or two hundred pairs of lungs, and
the impurities that arise from a leaky, overheated stove or furnace.   The time not devoted
to study is occupied in recitations, or exercises
that require a considerable degree of mental
activity.   To accomplish all the tasks, the regular school-hours are seldom sufficient, and more
or less time must be given to study out of
school.   It may be a single hour; it may be

two, three, or four. The time will be determined by the amount of the tasks; by the ambition, capacity, or excessive anxiety of the pupil.
With quick-witted children, who have no very
strong desire to excel, and those who have
neither desire nor capacity to excel, it is short.
On the contrary, with the sluggish but conscientious intellects, — with the ambitious who strive
for distinction, and the morbidly sensitive and
timid, — it is long. However this may be, it is
none the less a veritable fact, that in New England, to go no farther, more or less study out of
school is the general rule for all except the very
youngest scholars. This has been sometimes
questioned, if not positively denied, upon some
show of authority, perhaps, but on very unsatis-
factory grounds. The statements of a host of
parents who must be supposed to know something of the occupations of their children at
home, and of physicians whose professional duties often oblige them to make careful inquiry
on this subject, would seem to leave nothing
wanting in proof of our assertion. If particular
facts are required, nothing can be better than the
actual lessons, which will furnish every one
the means of judging for himself whether the
tasks can be accomplished in school. Here are
the lessons for a single day, given out not long
since, in a public school, to a class of girls

from twelve to fifteen years old. I have no reason to doubt that it is a fair specimen of the
daily work of the class. I mention no names,
because they are immaterial to the point in
hand :—

In Leach and Swan's Arithmetic, the 13th, 14th, and 15th
examples on the 181st page, and four extemporary.

In Greene's First-Lessons in Grammar, the 149th page as
far as the 6th sentence, to analyze.

In Smith's Quarto Geography, the Physical Geography of
Europe.

In Leach's Spelling-Book, the 59th and 60th pages, [con-
taining 162 words of two or three syllables.]

School-times 6 hours; average time occupied in recitations, 2 hours.

Here, again, is a day's work, taken at random,
of a more advanced class of girls, from fourteen
to seventeen :—

In Brockelsby's Astronomy, about 2 pages.

In Davies's Geometry, the 8th, 9th, and 10th propositions
of the Fourth Book.

In Poitevin's French Grammar, one page and ten verbs.

An exercise in composition once a fortnight.

School-time, 5 hours; time occupied in recitations, from
$2\frac{1}{2}$ to 3 hours; in general exercises and recesses, 1 hour.

The following were the lessons for a single
day, assigned to a class of boys from twelve to
fifteen years old :—

In Sherwin's Algebra, the 5th section.

In Worcester's History, one page in advance and two re-
viewed.

In Fasquelle's French Course, lesson 12th ; review, exercise 13th, three irregular verbs.

School-time, 6 hours.

These may be considered as average examples of the amount of work now put upon the youthful brain. They are the first that came to hand, but I have reason to believe that additional statistics of this kind would oftener show a larger than a smaller requirement. They will enable every one to judge for himself, with sufficient accuracy, whether the strain to which they subject the mind is or is not compatible with the highest degree of healthy endurance. In the first example, there is required, out of school, according to the statement of one of the class, a girl of average intellect, about two hours of study a day — sometimes more and sometimes less — making an aggregate of eight hours. In the second, the time given to study out of school is estimated by one of the class, standing at or near its head, to be from three to four hours. In the third, the history and the French are studied out of school. How much time this would take, any one may judge for himself.

In connection with this matter of out-of-school study, it must be considered that much of it is pursued in the evening, often until a late hour — a practice more pernicious to the health,

in youth or adult, than any other description of
mental exercise. The brain is in no condition
for sleep immediately after such occupation.
The mind is swarming with verbs and fractions
and triangles, and a tedious hour or two must
pass away before it falls into a restless, scarcely
refreshing slumber. Jaded and dispirited, it
enters upon the duties of the day with little of
that buoyancy which comes only from " nature's
sweet restorer."

Thus it is that, in all our cities and populous
villages, the tender mind is kept in a state of
the highest activity and effort, six or eight hours
a day, for several years in succession, with only
such intervals of rest as are furnished by the
weekly holiday and the occasional vacation.
Sunday can hardly be admitted among these
intervals, for that day also has its special school,
with its lessons and rewards. In other words,
it is subjected to an amount of task-work, which,
estimated merely by the time it requires, is
greater than what may be considered a proper
allowance to a cultivated, adult mind. Among
the easier classes of our people, the work of
education is accomplished, to a considerable
degree, in boarding-schools. Here, the inducements are stronger, perhaps, than in the public
schools, to go over the greatest possible extent
of ground. The pupils are somewhat advanced,

the terms are high, and much is expected from the outlay. Numerous attainments and brilliant accomplishments, rather than sound learning and good mental discipline, might naturally be expected under such circumstances, and such, I apprehend, is the ordinary result. Especially is this the case in schools for girls, on whom, with their more susceptible nervous organization, the system inflicts far more mischief than on the hardier nature of boys. In all our larger cities are fashionable schools, to which the daughters of the opulent families resort to obtain the finishing touches of what is called their education. The work must be accomplished speedily, for they are in haste, dropping forever all thoughts of study and instruction, to taste the pleasures of society.

The daily routine of one of this class of schools is exhibited in the following statement furnished by a pupil. The girls rise at six. Prayers at seven, and then study till eight. Breakfast. From nine to three, in school with fifteen minutes of recess. Dinner. Walk. One hour's study. One hour's recreation. Supper at seven. From eight to nine, study. Prayers and to bed. Other schools of a similar class present but little difference in regard to the amount of study and of recreation.

In villages and smaller towns may be found

another class of boarding-schools designed for a different description of girls, in which the useful is supposed to predominate over the ornamental. The amount of study, however, seems to be greater than in the more fashionable schools. In one of them, I find the daily exercises, as follows. The girls rise at half past five; put rooms in order; breakfast; study from seven till nine; school from nine till twelve; then dinner; after which relaxation till half past two, when school begins and continues till five; walk in the open air, or calisthenics in doors, till tea; study from seven till nine; prayers, and to bed at ten.

The following communication, entitled, by the young lady who sent it, *Life in a Boarding-School*, displays more exactly the manner in which the time of the pupils is occupied. " We rose at half past five. At six, one of the room-mates went to the parlor to study, while the other remained in her room until half past six, devoting the time ostensibly to meditation. At a quarter before seven, we breakfasted, and then put our rooms in order. At half past seven, those who studied before breakfast went to their rooms for meditation, while the others, who had meditated at that time, now studied half an hour. From eight till fifteen minutes before nine, all were obliged to study. From nine till twelve we were in school, with fifteen minutes' recess. Dinner at half past twelve, and study from a quarter after one to a quarter before two. At two went into school again, and stayed till half past four or five, — I cannot remember which, — with fifteen minutes' recess. The time till eight was given to recreation, tea included. From eight till nine the two 'half hours' were spent by the room-mates in the same way as before breakfast, each girl going to her room alone. At a quarter after nine we went to bed, and at half past nine every light was put out, and not a word, even in a whisper, was to be spoken after that. Saturday was mostly a holiday. In the morning we had the two 'half hours,' and then an hour and a half for study. After that until dinner we were obliged to remain in our rooms to attend to our wardrobe, &c. The afternoon was entirely our own. We could walk, drive, and do what we pleased. The evening was spent like other evenings. Sunday was anything but a day of rest for us. We rose half an hour later than on other mornings, and then had our 'half hour' as usual. Until church-time we studied harder than on any other day in the week. All were obliged to attend service. We dined as soon as we got back from service, and then studied half an hour. After the afternoon service, we recited

9

the Bible lesson for which we had been preparing during the day. After tea, they had prayer-meetings in many of the rooms. From eight till nine, the two 'half hours' again. Those who remained in the parlor were obliged to give an abstract of the sermons. During the study-hours, as well as school-time, we were not allowed to speak a word. As for talking, we quite forgot there was such an art, as out of the twenty-four hours there were only about five when we were allowed to speak to one another."

The small proportion of time given to exercise and recreation, as indicated in these accounts, is a noteworthy fact, because it is signally short of what the whole system craves and needs, even under ordinary circumstances. If anything can counteract the exhaustive effects of intellectual occupation during eight or ten hours in the day, in young, growing girls, it is a liberal allowance of exhilarating exercise and recreation. The little which forms a part of the boarding-school routine is not exhilarating, and therefore needs an essential element of what it should be. Neither is it a liberal allowance, for it usually consists of a stiff, formal walk in the public street or road, for an hour or less, when the weather permits, without any end or object beyond that of mere locomotion. Of

one school, it was said that "in bad weather
they go into ·a narrow room in the basement,
and keep themselves warm by jumping about,
or hovering around a stove."

When it is considered too that, in addition to
all this systematic mismanagement, the girls
often sleep in crowded, ill-ventilated dormitories;
that their food is poor, and vitiated by all
the abominations of American cookery; that
their meals are taken hurriedly, twenty minutes
only being allowed for dinner, in one instance;
it ought not to be a matter of surprise, that so
many of them finally become pale, languid,
nervous, and hysterical.

Bad as all this is, we often hear of mental
exercises imposed upon students that are positively frightful. The lapse of nearly fifty
years has failed to obliterate from my own mind
an uneasy remembrance of weariness and distress occasioned by the effort of committing to
memory, for a Sunday lesson, many a dreary
page of the " Assembly's Catechism." In fact,
no faculty of the mind is so sorely pressed in
all our schools as that of memory, for the reason, no doubt, that the results are more readily
appreciated than those which come from any
other kind of intellectual discipline. The following statement would be almost incredible
were it not made on unquestionable authority.
" In the school in which I was educated [Win-

chester], it was the custom once a year that boys in the middle and lower classes should repeat all the Latin and Greek poetry they had learned in the year, with such additions to it of fresh matter as each boy could accomplish. So much did our place in the school depend on success in this, and so severe was the rivalry, that although we were then only about fourteen years of age, the usual quantity for the boys to repeat was from six to eight thousand lines, which we did in eight different lessons, and it took about a week to hear us. One boy, in my year, construed and repeated the enormous quantity of fourteen thousand lines of Homer, Horace, and Virgil; I heard him say it; the master dodged him about very much, but he scarcely ever missed a single word. One wonders in what chamber of the brain it could possibly have been stored away.

"Now I do not think that this excessive strain on the mnemonic faculty is calculated to strengthen it; nor do I believe that this or any other faculty ought to be so severely pressed. I have a lively recollection of the long-sustained exertion it required; how, week after week, we rose early, and late took rest, in our anxiety to outstrip others, upon which our station in the school, and, I may say, the *bread* of many of us depended." *

* Fearon. *What to learn and What to unlearn.* Lond. 1860. p. 93.

Let us now look at the effects of this immoderate mental effort on the health of the
mind. No doubt the greater part of the pupils
go through the process without any appreciable damage whatever. They proceed from
one study to another, rapidly accumulating their
acquisitions, and finish by knowing a little of
everything, and no one can point out any impairment of their physical or mental health.
From this it is too readily inferred that hard
study is quite innocent of the mischief we attribute to it. We might as well ignore the danger of cholera or diphtheria, because the great
majority of the community escape their attacks.
Whether this kind of discipline is best calculated to promote the future vigor and efficiency
of the mind, is another and a very important
question, which it forms no part of my present
purpose to discuss. Upon a portion of the scholars — comparatively small, no doubt, though
larger than it is generally supposed — it is just
as unquestionably disastrous. The proximate
causes of this result are various. These youths
may not have possessed the stamina of others;
their nervous system may have been unusually
irritable; or some moral motive may have induced them to prolong the hours of study to a
limit beyond the power of the stoutest constitution to bear. However this may be, there

remains the stubborn fact, that, in one way or another, they are suffering from excessive mental application.

The manner in which the evil is manifested is not very uniform, but however various the results, they agree in the one essential element of a disturbed or diminished nervous energy. It rarely comes immediately in the shape of insanity, for that is not a disease of childhood or early youth. It impairs the power of concentrating the faculties and of mastering difficult problems, every attempt thereat producing confusion and distress. It banishes the hope and buoyancy natural to youth, and puts in their place anxiety, gloom, and apprehension. It diminishes the conservative power of the animal economy, to such a degree, that attacks of disease, which otherwise would have passed off safely, destroy life almost before danger is anticipated. Every intelligent physician understands that, other things being equal, the chances of recovery are far less in the studious, highly intellectual child, than in one of an opposite description. Among the more obvious and immediate effects upon the nervous system, are unaccountable restlessness, disturbed and deficient sleep, loss of appetite, epilepsy, chorea, and especially a kind of irritability and exhaustion, which leads the van of a host of other ills, bodily and mental, that seriously impair the efficiency and comfort of the individual.

I have said that insanity is rarely an immediate effect of hard study at school, but I do not doubt that it lays the foundation of many a later attack. When a person becomes insane, people look around for the cause of his affliction, and fix upon the most recent event apparently capable of producing it. *Post hoc propter hoc,* is the common philosophy on such occasions. But if the whole mental history of the patient were clearly unfolded to our view, we should often find, I apprehend, at a much earlier period, some agency far more potent in causing the evil, than the misfortune, or the passion, or the bereavement, or the disappointment, which attracts the common attention. Among these remoter agencies in the production of mental disease, I doubt if any one, except hereditary defects, is more common, at the present time, than excessive application of the mind when young. The immediate mischief may have seemed slight, or have readily disappeared after a total separation from books and studies, aided, perhaps, by change of scene; but the brain is left in a condition of peculiar impressibility which renders it morbidly sensitive to every adverse influence.

The precise period at which school instruction should begin will vary a little, of course, in dif-

ferent children; but I feel quite safe in saying
that it should seldom be until the sixth or seventh year. Not that the mind should be kept in
a state of inactivity until this time, for that is
impossible. It will necessarily be receiving impressions from the external world, and these will
begin the work of stimulating and unfolding its
various faculties. Instinctively the young child
seeks for knowledge of some kind, and its spontaneous efforts may be safely allowed. With
a little management, indeed, they may be made
subservient to very important acquisitions. In
the same way that it learns the names of its
toys and playthings, it may learn the names of
its letters, of geometrical figures, and objects of
natural history. There can be but little danger
of such exercises being carried too far. But the
discipline of school, of obliging the tender child
to sit upright on an uncomfortable seat, for several hours in the day, and con his lessons from
a book, is dangerous both to mind and body.
To the latter, because it craves exercise almost
incessantly, and suffers pain, if not distortion,
from its forced quietude and unnatural postures.
To the former, because it is pleased with tran-
sient emotions, and seeks for a variety of impressions calculated to gratify its perceptive
faculties. The idea of *study* considered in relation to the infant mind, of appropriating and

assimilating the contents of a book, of performing mental processes that require a considerable
degree of attention and abstraction, indicates an
ignorance of the real constitution of the infant
mind that would be simply ridiculous, did it not
lead to pain, weariness, and disgust. And such
is the strange abandonment of all practical common sense on this subject, that many a person
fails to view this practice in its true light, who
would never commit the folly of beginning the
training of a colt by taking it from the side of
its dam, harnessing it to a cart or plough, and
keeping it at work through a sultry summer's
day.

At the age of six or seven, then, the child may
be sent to school, or have its stated tasks. This
period may be very properly anticipated in some
cases, and delayed in others, but practically it
will not be found expedient to vary from it
much. Children of quick and mature minds
may accomplish much before this age, but such
minds should be held in check, rather than stimulated to exertion, and more dull and sluggish
intellects should, for that very reason, begin their
training without farther delay. The process of
education, it must be considered, makes large
drafts on the physical powers. Confinement to
the benches of a schoolroom for several hours in
the day, accompanied by close application of

the mind, is a very different thing from the un-
restrained use of the limbs and powers of locomotion, and careless rambling of the attention,
so natural to youth. A firm and robust child,
of a sanguine temperament, will obviously meet
the demand on his vital powers better than the
thin, lymphatic, tenderly nurtured child whom
the winds of heaven have not been allowed to
visit too roughly. I fear these physical diversities have not been sufficiently considered by
teachers, in regulating the mental discipline of
their pupils; for the medical man has frequent
occasion to deplore, without being able to remedy, the mischief that arises from inattention to
this fact. In regard to the character of the individual mind in this relation, it need merely
be said, that, if characterized by quickness and
aptitude, it will bear a somewhat greater amount
of exercise than one of an opposite character;
but the risk of overworking a mind of the
former temper is sufficient to deter us from
increasing its tasks.

CHAPTER III.

MENTAL HYGIENE AS AFFECTED BY MENTAL CONDITIONS AND INFLUENCES.

WE come now to consider a class of agencies
more or less affecting the health of the mind,
which are exclusively mental. In a great degree they are under our control, and it depends
upon ourselves — upon our enlightenment and
resolution — whether they are made instru-
ments of good or of evil. It depends very
much upon ourselves whether we so manage
our minds, that every exercise will add something to their capacity and vigor, or only detract
from their energies, defeat their original purposes, and lead to a feeble, if not manifestly
morbid, result. Owing probably to the disposition to regard the mind as an indivisible principle, too little account has been made of its
diversities, tendencies, and aptitudes, its susceptibility to outward influences, and its power,
within certain limits, of modifying its manifestations. Philosophers lay down rules for the
conduct of the understanding, and sages mark
out the path which leads to virtue and happi-

ness. But something more is needed to enable
the mind to act efficiently, and to increase its
capacity for labor and endurance. Many a
man may assent to the precepts of Locke and
Watts, whose whole mental training is calculated to nullify their teaching, and lead to a
lame and impotent result. The problem presented to every child of Adam is this, — having
received certain powers of mind from nature,
how are they to be managed so as to insure the
greatest possible return? Observe, it is not how
he may succeed in writing a good poem, or
making a great bargain, or creating a sensation,
but how he can keep his mind at the working-
point in every department of effort, whether
that effort be poetry or philosophy, or the common business of life, and in such a manner that
its exercise be not hampered by debility or
disease.

In order to maintain the highest degree of
mental vigor, it is necessary that every power
which nature has bestowed shall have its rightful share of influence in the habitual experience
of the individual. I do not mean that every
power is to be cultivated alike, and that no particular one is to preponderate in the moral or intellectual character. But every power is given
us for wise and good purposes, and if any one
is so entirely neglected that it might as well

have never existed, or, worse still, so perverted
as to minister to a very different end, then an
element of strength is lost. The faculties and
sentiments are not entirely distinct and independent of one another, although, if we choose,
they may be cultivated and developed as if they
had no very intimate connection. Much of our
mental activity and mental training is exceedingly partial, that is, confined to a few of the
powers, the rest being scarcely exercised at all,
or remaining completely dormant. This kind
of management is supposed to be required by
the social condition of the race ; and, no doubt,
if judiciously applied, with the qualifications incident to every general principle, it will insure
a desirable result. But it may now be received
as a settled truth, that no power of the mind
can be entirely neglected without detriment to
some of the rest. With all their independence,
they stand in need of the check and correction
and enforcement of one another. As well might
the eye say unto the hand, I have no need of
thee, or the head say to the feet, I have no need
of you, as the ideal power say to that which investigates causes and effects, I have no need of
thee, or the religious sentiment say to the benevolent sentiment, I have no need of thee.

No man can measure his own capacities, nor
apply them to the best possible use, whose pow-

ers have been very unequally cultivated. His mind will present a one-sided and imperfect character, wanting that full and rounded development which is necessary to practical achievement in the great purposes of life. Men of this stamp may dazzle, and even astonish, but they accomplish little. Whatever form of mental activity they may display, they are apt to be led away by it into the pursuit of unprofitable schemes instead of directing it to fruitful results. It may even get beyond control altogether, and then begins to be morbid. Besides, if, under pretence of concentrating himself upon a particular pursuit, a person neglects everything else capable of furnishing occupation to a rational mind, and loses his interest in whatever else most men regard as important or worthy of consideration, he is in danger, not only of frustrating the very object he is after, but of losing entirely the healthy balance of his faculties. Much of the unhappiness of men arises from the fault in question, for the intellectual cultivation and exercise to which they had looked as a means of social elevation and material prosperity, only lead to failure and disappointment.

Our limits will not admit of a very copious illustration of this point, and therefore we must be content with a few instances among the most common and significant.

One of the most prolific sources of mental inefficiency in this our day and generation, is the undue cultivation of that power which, under one name or another, is chiefly occupied with conceptions of the beautiful, the exquisite, and whatever else is calculated to please the taste, excite emotion, or gratify and charm the fancy. No form of intellectual activity is so common as this. Under all degrees of refinement, — in sage or savage, idolater or saint, child or man, — it is equally obvious, varying only in the objects to which it is applied. In all, it relieves the hard, dull monotony of real life with inexhaustible sources of excitement and recreation. In youth and health and innocence, it gilds the future with the warmest tints of joy and hope, and invests every scene that it creates with a charm peculiarly its own. In disease its normal functions may be so disturbed that the conceptions become cheerless and painful beyond the experience of reality, and are bodied forth with a distinctness more vivid and terrible than any mere object of sense could present. In youth, especially, is this faculty active; and one of the crying faults of the education of our times is that it encourages its exercise to a degree incompatible with the claims of the other faculties. The license of youth is seldom corrected by the wisdom of riper years, and the whole mental history of the individual betrays the influence of this single fault. It begets a distaste for exact knowledge, for that is the fruit of laborious study; it indisposes the mind to habits of continuous thought, and quenches all thirst for intellectual excellence. The pleasures of the imagination are always accessible, and they can be enjoyed with little of that preparation which is needed in the case of other intellectual pleasures. This would be bad enough did the evil stop here, but it extends much farther. It actually incapacitates the individual for those intellectual efforts that are required for the great purposes of life, and circumscribes the sphere in which he can move with any degree of credit to himself or good to others. An imagination thus indulged, and feeling none of those checks and balances which the cultivation of other faculties would afford, easily wanders into devious paths that lead at last to helpless and hopeless derangement. Life becomes a dream, and that dream needs only favoring circumstances to be converted into delusion. I think it may be stated as one of the results of modern observation, that the man who enters upon life with no habits of serious and connected thought, with no taste for investigating the causes and effects of the countless phenomena passing around him, with no practical object clearly set before him and worthy the pursuit of a rational creature, whose joys and sorrows, whose principles and motives, whose ends and aims, are fashioned by the plastic touch of his own busy imagination, cannot promise himself exemption from mental disease, if at all predisposed thereto.

Even where this exclusive cultivation of the ideal power is manifested in a devotion to poetry or the fine arts, the actual performance will always evince imperfections that spring from the neglect of the other faculties. The great poet or painter is far from being a man of one idea. He achieves his position, not more by the flights of his fancy, than by the wisdom that informs and animates his ideas. The Plays of Shakspeare abound with the practical sagacity of Bacon's Essays; the grandeur of Milton is derived, in no small degree, from his rich and varied learning; Leonardo, Michael Angelo, Raphael, sounded the depths of philosophy, and their immortal works bear many a trace of their large and liberal culture.

The mischievous consequences of having but one idea are still more obvious where this idea springs from some over-stimulated sentiment or affection. A person's mind becomes strongly fixed, for instance, on his religious obligations, and he scarcely thinks of anything else. The af-

fairs of his fellow-creatures, and the great events
of the time, are regarded as vanity of vani-
ties when compared with the momentous concerns that engross his attention. At all times
and on all occasions, he dwells upon the favorite
theme, and wonders that others should not do
like him. In short, the religious sentiment in
such a person is divorced entirely from its
proper relations to his fellow-men, and becomes
a purely selfish emotion. The evil that flows
from this condition varies with the mental constitution of those who manifest it, but in all it
is deplorable, and has furnished some of the
saddest chapters in the history of the race. In
some it is an overweening confidence in their
own religious condition, which may not always
be allied to correct conduct. In some it is a
rabid fanaticism, that shuts the heart against
the claims of God and humanity; that delivers
them up an easy prey to the arts of unprincipled
and crafty men, and precipitates them, perhaps,
upon a career of pitiable extravagance and folly.
In others it consists in distorted views of religious truth, in excessive hopes or fears, in
painful apprehensions and forebodings, and,
finally, in fixed, it may be incurable, delusion.
And thus it happens that a sentiment, intended,
beyond all others, when properly trained and
regulated, to promote the present and future

happiness of man, is turned into a source of un-
utterable woe.

The sentiment of benevolence, allying us, as
it does, to the great Giver of all good, would
seem, at first thought, less likely than any other
to be the source of an unhealthy activity; and
yet when so strong as to be the predominant
trait in the moral constitution, it is liable, in the
class of cases under consideration, if not carefully watched, to lead to the most painful results. When thus indulged, life, duty, right and
wrong, God and man, are often viewed solely
by the light of this sentiment, with none of
those softening shadows which the rest, under a
more equal cultivation, would impart. Justice,
discretion, expediency, even right, must all
yield to the mere impulses of benevolence,
which recognize no degrees nor shades in moral
obligation. Oppression under any and every
form must be immediately abated by an appeal
to force; reforms are to be thrust upon the
world, regardless of time or season; abuses are
to be torn up by the roots, careless of the
healthy growth around that may be injured by
the process; and individuals are held to be responsible for any wrong with which they may
be ever so remotely connected. Whatever is,
is absolutely right or absolutely wrong, to be
fondly cherished or summarily destroyed. No

palliation of the evil is to be found in the attending circumstances ; no remedy is to be tolerated that implies any prospective change in the delinquent. Thus, it becomes, at last, to be regarded as a sacred duty to vindicate the claims of abstract benevolence at whatever hazard, even though it lead through seas of blood and fire. Let those who thus allow their benevolent sentiments to shape their conduct and opinions reflect that, little as they may suspect it, every day is bearing them beyond the reach of those healthful activities which prevent eccentric movements of the mind from passing over the limits of safety.

Time would fail to illustrate the many ways in which this exclusive cultivation of a single power impairs the efficiency of the mind. The fact itself cannot be doubted, and the reason is sufficiently obvious. It does not imply, however, that every power should be equally cultivated, for this would be impracticable in the nature of things. But it does imply that every power, having been implanted within us for a necessary purpose, should be enabled, by a judicious conduct of the mind, to furnish its rightful share in the formation of the moral and intellectual character.

A partial cultivation of the mental faculties is incompatible, not only with the highest order of thought, but with the highest degree of health and efficiency. The results of professional experience fairly warrant the statement, that in persons of a high grade of intellectual endowment and cultivation, other things being equal, the force of moral shocks is more easily broken, tedious and harassing exercises of particular powers more safely borne, than in those of an opposite description; and disease, when it comes, is more readily controlled and cured. The kind of management which consists in awakening a new order of emotions, in exciting new trains of thought, in turning attention to some new matter of study or speculation, must be far less efficacious, because less applicable, in one whose mind has always had a limited range, than in one of larger resources and capacities. In endeavoring to restore the disordered mind of the clodhopper, who has scarcely an idea beyond that of his manual employment, the great difficulty is to find some available point from which conservative influences may be projected. He dislikes reading, he never learned amusements, he feels no interest in the affairs of the world, and unless the circumstances allow of some kind of bodily labor, his mind must remain in a state of solitary isolation, brooding over its morbid fancies, and utterly incompetent to initiate any recuperative movement.

There are many persons in the world endowed
by nature with what may be called ill-balanced
minds — some faculties or sentiments being ex-
cessively or deficiently developed, and thus preventing that coöperation and harmony of action
necessary to the best results. The particular
form which this sort of endowment may assume
differs in different cases, and therefore cannot be
generally described, but an instance or two will
furnish a sufficiently correct idea of my meaning.

In some it is manifested in a want of admin-
istrative ability, or practical discernment. They
have, apparently, good intellectual powers, they
think vigorously and clearly, their plans are
specious and comprehensive. They may be not
without considerable knowledge of men, and
some familiarity with the ways of the world.
They may possess some force of will and energy
of purpose, with a strong desire and determina-
tion to excel. By those whose knowledge of
character is not very profound, these men are
regarded as eminently calculated to succeed in
their undertakings, — an opinion not justified
by the result. When the opportunity for action
arrives, — when called on to apply their faculties
to some practical purpose, — the mental defect
appears, and they lamentably fail. The true
relation between the idea elaborated in the mind

and the idea embodied in actual form, between
the conception and the execution, the project
and the performance, is not clearly discerned,
and the strongest effort results in an impotent
beating of the air. The right thing is done at
the wrong time, or in the wrong place; the
sagacious plan is carried into execution under
circumstances incompatible with success; the
master-stroke is delivered with a feeble hand, or
an uncertain aim; the favorable moment, the
fortunate contingency, is unobserved, or observed too late. In short, the career of this class
of persons presents an unbroken series of disappointments and failures. When, to this kind of
mental endowment, there is joined an overweening estimate of one's own capacities, the
result is still more disastrous, because more is
attempted. Unable to discern the limits of their
ability, these persons are apt to presume beyond
the measure of a safe confidence, and are ever
ready to attribute their failure to any other than
the true source.

There is another class, who, with talents adequate to almost anything, seem born to accomplish nothing. Their ends may be worthy and
well-defined, their aspirations pure and lofty,
and their industry unflagging; but their career
is determined rather by some adventitious circumstances than by the essential conditions of

the objects which they have placed before them. In a word, they are governed by fancy rather than judgment, and thus are led about by every *ignis fatuus* that comes in their way. They have no sooner made some perceptible progress towards their object than their attention is diverted to more attractive paths, which are ardently pursued for a season, to be, in their turn, abandoned the moment the gloss of novelty is lost. Discovering often that they have mistaken their mission, they go through life, ever seeking, never finding it. They are ever on the verge of some grand discovery or brilliant achievement which always eludes their grasp, for lack of that unfaltering purpose, that concentrated effort which alone will insure success. The very intensity of their conceptions blinds them to whatever is not directly before them, and, failing to see what everybody else sees, they are all the more confident in themselves, and less disposed to heed the suggestions of others.

Sometimes the imperfect balance of the mind arises from excessive or deficient development in the moral powers, with a result still more deplorable to the individual and to the world. Some men, for instance, go on from the cradle to the grave, with only the most imperfect perception of those great moral distinctions which are obvious enough to most men of the same race and period. With them right and wrong are merely conventional terms, expressive of some relation to their immediate interests; honor, honesty, integrity, only indicate a quality of character that may or may not be desirable, according to circumstances; and duplicity, deceit, calumny, are only justifiable weapons in fighting the battle of life. This moral trait is not the result of bad education or extraordinary temptations, but of a natural defect, which disqualifies its possessor from discerning the immutable, independent existence of right and wrong, virtue and vice, just as another defect prevents some persons from distinguishing colors. It not unfrequently appears in connection with great intellectual powers, and even strong religious sensibilities; and then, if the individual does not prove to be a pest to the world, it is only because of some happy concurrence of circumstances, which clearly renders the practice of virtue in some degree necessary to the furtherance of his own ends. These facts enable us to account for the conflicting opinions that have been passed on many a man who has made his mark on the times. They teach us why the same character, according as he is regarded from different points of view, or by different kinds of persons, may be deemed by one as both good and great, and by another as only selfish and cunning.

Again, the moral defect may consist in an undue estimate of one's abilities. Some persons believe themselves competent to any thing to which their reckless ambition may aspire, and lay their plans on a scale of grandeur utterly beyond their reach. To question their preten- sions is to provoke their wrath, and make them enemies for life. Of course, they often exhibit a lamentable disproportion between their prom- ise and their performance; failure waits upon every move, and they end with being the con- tempt of men, who, endowed with far less abilities, better know their measure, and what they are capable of doing.

The passions, too, may be so inordinately developed as to impair the efficiency and hap- piness of the individual. Some persons for instance, with all the force of an instinct, view whatever passes around them with a jealous eye, —ever ready to find in the sayings and doings of others evidence of hostility or unfriendliness, and to see in the most trivial occurrences matured designs of annoyance. They are constantly breaking with their best friends, and spend their whole lives in converting the innocent occasions of private and public intercourse into pretexts for coldness and disaffection. Others are unfitted for happiness and usefulness by excessive envy. Their blessings, whether small or great, are of little satisfaction, because others are enjoying what seem to them still greater. Favors bestowed on others are regarded as proofs of the most culpable neglect of their own superior deserts. They feel as if every one who has any reason to rejoice in the good things of life were guilty of a positive wrong towards them, and bound to make restitution and recompense.

It would be needless to multiply illustrations of the *ill-balanced* mind. Sufficient has been said to establish the fact, and exhibit its importance in this connection. Such defects of nature can never be entirely remedied, but early judicious discipline and persistent self-control may do much to repress their growth and counteract their effects. This implies the highest function of education, and one too much overlooked in an age which requires of the teacher only to fill the mind of the pupil with various knowledge. It is well to bear in mind, too, that these defects not only impair the mental efficiency, but they are indicative of morbid tendencies which may be easily converted into positive disease, — a result which only the highest prudence in the conduct of life and the most skilful managment of the mind, will effectually prevent.

Man, as a social animal, is endowed with

the faculties necessary for bringing him into relation with his fellow-men. They are bound together, not merely by that community of interests which is discovered by a process of reasoning, but by an intuitive sense of the emotions which agitate the breast and determine the conduct and happiness of the individual. A principle more prompt and impulsive than the slow and cautious deductions of reason is required to meet all the exigences of the social state; and its existence, in some of its forms at least, has long been recognized under the names of *sympathy* and *propensity to imitate.* It is in ceaseless operation wherever men are gathered together; but whether quietly and irresistibly upon scattered individuals, or with tremendous manifestations of its power upon large masses, few are aware of its nature — many, not even of its existence — and fewer still apprehend the importance of rightly regulating its influence upon themselves. Education, habit, temperament may affect its operation, but cannot eradicate it. The conditions on which it depends are imperfectly understood, and its effects are regarded with the same kind of surprise and curiosity with which we witness the most strange and unexpected phenomena of nature.

The principle in question has been too much

considered as a supplementary element in our mental constitution, manifesting itself in curious and anomalous phenomena rather than as an all-pervading, indispensable principle, without which the great ends of our being would utterly fail. It needs no profound knowledge of the springs of human action to perceive that every man's daily experience reveals, in some way or other, the operation of this law of our nature. Indeed it can hardly be questioned that, in populous communities, it determines, more than anything else, not only those great social movements which possess an historical importance, but also the sentiments and impulses which, for good or for ill, shape the views and conduct of the individual. Independent, self-originating movement is, probably, a far rarer thing than that which springs, more or less directly, from some outward source, which is to be found in the prevailing mental movements that, like the atmosphere about us, exert an increasing, unconscious, inevitable pressure. If these are distinguished by disordered imagination, by grovelling propensities, by unhallowed desires, their ultimate influence on the individual mind will be devoid of every element of good. By an irresistible and inevitable law, they impart their own moral complexion to whatever they involve in their progress. The teachings of the school and

the church, and the precepts of philosophy and
religion have much to do, no doubt, with shap-
ing the character and conduct of men; but the
thoughts, emotions, and impulses awakened by
the mental movements around them are often
the efficient forces that determine the great
events of life. To learn what a man will do
in a given social emergency, we must look, not
only to his special training and the prominent
qualities of his character, but also to the cur-
rents of feeling in which he moves and the tone
of thought which prevails around him. The
secret springs and forces of society are to be
sought for, not in the treatises of morality and
philosophy that happen to be in vogue, but in
the newspaper, the pamphlet, the novel, the
song, where, without concert or mutual understanding, are displayed the objects and aspirations by which large masses of men are swayed.
In this way is revealed the hygienic condition
of the popular mind, between which and the
nutriment it craves, there must always exist a
very close relation. The ephemeral literature
of a people will always indicate, therefore, the
degree of mental strength, efficiency, and endurance, to which the people have attained. And
it is in the moral atmosphere which they habitually breathe that we may find the forces
which upheave the passions and quicken all

the pulses of their being, rather than in the
occasional influences that act directly and spe-
cially on the individual.

This view of the subject has been too little
considered, for though it may be admitted in
general terms, its practical application has always been very defective. In looking for the
origin of insanity, we are too apt to confine
our attention to the class of influences which
lie near at hand and directly before our face,
and fail to discern those agencies which, though
more remote and obscure, may be none the less
efficient. The bereavement or misfortune which
apparently drove reason from her throne may
have had less to do with this result than the
habitual train of thought and emotion which
supplies the mind with no additional power,
but rather diminishes its energies by its fruitless activities. In regard to this latter class of
agencies, the mind is governed very much by
the law of sympathy. The deductions of reason are deliberately wrought out, every man
working for himself, while sympathetic movements, even of the deepest character, are propagated with a kind of electric rapidity.

The operation of this law may be witnessed
in the daily life and habitual conduct of men.
Any mental movement that can be manifested
by sensible signs, excites in some degree a cor-

responding movement in others. We are instinctively impelled — some more, some less, strongly — to imitate whatever others are feeling and doing around us. The passion or emotion exhibited by one excites the same passion or emotion in others, as a musical sound puts into vibration certain chords in its neighborhood, and thus is propagated to an indefinite extent. Whoever lives in close communion with one who is irascible, peevish, and overbearing, is liable to become equally irascible and peevish, unless prevented by a large endowment of restraining grace. The sad, depressed, and sorrowing spirit will inevitably impart its leaden tinge to all who live within its shadow. The hopeful, the trusting, the strong, infuse their hope and strength into others, by the mere force of example; while the visionary, scheming, castle-building enthusiast unconsciously spreads the roseate hues of his own atmosphere over the humbler conceptions of his neighbor. In like manner, forbearance, gentleness, love, and kindness shed forth their genial influences in actual life, with more certainty of their taking root and abiding, than when formally inculcated in lessons of morality and religion.

The instinctive propensity to imitate is manifested, as already intimated, irrespective of the qualities of the thing imitated, and to such a degree as to overpower the tendencies of culture and of grace. When the poet said,

"Vice is a monster of such hideous mien,
That to be hated needs but to be seen,"

he disregarded the fact that, under certain conditions of the nervous system, nothing is too monstrous to excite a feeling of sympathy leading to imitation. Then murder, suicide, and other crimes, need only to be brought before the attention, in the shape of some actual example, especially if marked by striking incidents, in order to be repeated by many in whom, by reason of defective training, or morbid tendencies, whether congenital or acquired, or both combined, such narratives always touch some congenial chord. It is a great mistake to suppose that cases of flagrant delinquency are always regarded, even by persons not very deficient, apparently, in moral or intellectual endowments, with sentiments of loathing, or even as matters of curiosity, exciting only a transitory thought or emotion. The truth is, they often excite the very class of emotions in which these examples originated; and thus is accomplished the first step towards a repetition of similar acts. This result is produced in one of two ways: either directly, by touching some congenial spring in a mind prepared for it by morbid proclivities; or indirectly, by familiarizing

11

the mind with the aspects of vice, and thus blunting the original keenness of the moral perceptions. From one or the other of these causes, it happens that, in every community, there are multitudes ready to receive impressions that will, more or less seriously, derange their mental health. They are marked by no peculiarities ; they are supposed to be perfectly straight and sound, and when the disaster comes, it seems like thunder from a cloudless sky. It is this latent susceptibility to mental disorder which often renders the operation of the law of sympathy so pernicious, and converts an agency intended only to enlarge the sphere of our enjoyment, into an instrument of mischief and woe.

The law of sympathy is no less efficient in the propagation of tastes, aptitudes, and habits. Over and above the appeal made by every example to the reasoning faculties, there is an instinctive tendency to admire what others admire, to seek distinction where it is sought by others, to fall into the same social routine which is followed in the community around us. In this process of assimilation the intellect is entirely passive, and the result is accomplished without calculation, and almost unconsciously. The individual is transformed without being aware of the change.

The same effect may be witnessed in the propagation of intellectual and political movements. Of course, special attainments can be achieved only by special efforts, and great truths are the rewards obtained only by toiling, persevering genius. But the current opinions, the prevailing views, the general tone of thinking, which characterize the times and leave their mark on the fortunes of the race, are propagated more by sympathy than by those convictions that spring from elaborate investigation. Many, if not most of those remarkable movements which constitute epochs in the history of the race, were not effected, apparently, by a course of patient preparation and persevering endeavor. So little were they anticipated, so surprising did they seem, even to those who witnessed their occurrence, that men were more disposed to gaze on them with wonder, than to seek for their causes and conditions. It would seem, sometimes, as if a new thought need only to be uttered to arrest attention and be followed by speedy conviction and effort. Independent of any process of logic, or any arts of rhetoric, it meets a hearty response, while the public mind, before unruffled as a placid lake, heaves and swells under the unwonted impulse. The Reformation by Luther, and the revolutions in America and France, were not altogether the results of arguments carefully prepared and forcibly stated by the popular leaders, in favor of religious and political freedom, but, in a great degree, of those instantaneous and irresistible convictions which run from mind to mind with the rapidity of an electric flash. Such events can be explained upon no hypothesis that does not recognize the principle in question, though generally overlooked, or very inadequately estimated, in the popular philosophy.

Nothing shows more clearly the independence of this principle of any exercise of the will, than the fact that it sometimes involves the animal frame in its operation. The convulsions of hysteria, it is well known, are apt to be propagated among young women by force of imitation. The same trait has been observed in chorea, stammering, and other nervous affections. Boerhaave relates that the pupils of a squint-eyed schoolmaster, near Leyden, after a while, exhibited the same obliquity of vision. John Wesley, in describing the exercises of some of his converts, says that they were buffeted of Satan in an unusual manner, by such a spirit of laughter as they could in no wise resist, though it was pain and grief to them. He was the less surprised at it, he says, because he had himself experienced the same affection. One Sunday when he and his brother were walking in the fields and singing psalms, as was their custom, he (the brother) burst out into loud laughter. " I asked him if he were distracted, and began to be very angry, and, presently after, to laugh as loud as he. Nor could we possibly refrain, though we were ready to tear ourselves to pieces." *

It would be inconsistent with my present purpose, to recount those scenes, — seldom witnessed now, happily, but still too often for the credit of modern enlightenment, — where, favored by popular ignorance, religious fanaticism, and false philosophy, the principle in question has been exhibited on a large scale. In the fifteenth, sixteenth, and seventeenth centuries, in schools, convents, and secluded villages, they were of frequent occurrence, and characterized by many remarkable features. Beginning with a single individual, generally of the softer sex, the affection, whatever form it might take, rapidly spread through whole communities, and numbered its victims by scores and hundreds. Starting from some trivial nervous disturbance, it soon involved both the sensorial and muscular systems, and was manifested by every possible expression of abnormal activity. And it must ever remain one of the wonders of human pathology, how rude

* *Journal*, 9th May, 1740.

peasants, young girls, and even children, with no knowledge of the world, and no training whatever, could at once perform feats of muscular power beyond the reach of the accomplished gymnast, and imitate sounds and movements with the correctness of a professional actor. Anything beyond a brief allusion to some of these occurrences, our limits forbid.

At the beginning of the seventeenth century, some fourscore women in the commune of Amou, France, were seized with a strong convulsive affection, during which they rolled and tumbled about on the ground, striking their heads against whatever stood in the way, and their limbs against each other; and the united effort of three strong men was unable, on one occasion, to restrain the movement of a single arm. During the paroxysm, the most of them barked or howled like a dog; hence the disorder was called *mal de laïra*. In 1566, an orphan asylum in Amsterdam was the scene of one of these extraordinary affections. In the course of the paroxysm, the children would mew like a cat, climb trees, and run about the housetops, without falling or any other accident. An old writer relates that in a convent near Paris, a large number of the nuns were seized, every day at the same hour, with a remarkable nervous affection which set them all mewing, " to the great

scandal of religion." In 1642, one of those
forms of nervous disorder which it was the custom in those days to attribute to witchcraft,
prevailed in a convent in Louviers, France.
Among other convulsive movements which the
nuns exhibited was that of bending back in the
form of an arc until the head touched the floor,
— the body thus resting on the head and feet
only, and that without the help of the hands.

The *Trembleurs of Cevennes* — a sect of
French Protestants driven by persecution into
a state of gross fanaticism, towards the end of
the seventeenth century — preached and proph-
esied, while their bodily frame shook with a
strange agitation and trembling. Marshal Vil-
lars, who witnessed some scenes in this epidemic, says that in one town, every woman and
girl, without exception, appeared to be possessed by the devil. The *Convulsionnaires of
St. Medard*, as they were called, had only to lie
down on the tomb of a venerated deacon of
the church, — the Abbe Paris, whose remains
were supposed to shed forth a healing influence
upon bodily disease, — to be seized with the
most wonderful contortions of the neck, trunk,
and limbs, and often of limbs that had been
paralyzed for years. Among the thousands
thus affected were every description of persons, — professed devotees, sceptics, idlers,

Jesuits, the halt, the lame, the blind, and children of tender years.*

Never were such convulsive affections more extensively and curiously manifested than in the subjects of those great religious awakenings which agitated the Western States towards the beginning of the present century. The bodily exercises by which they were characterized were classed and named by a clerical writer of the time, as, first, the falling exercise; second, the jerking exercise; third, the rolling exercise; fourth, the running exercise; fifth, the dancing exercise; sixth, the barking exercise; seventh, the visions and trances. In these various exercises were embraced almost every possible combination of muscular movement, and the subjects of them were reckoned by hundreds and thousands. Of the jerking exercise, it is said, " His head was thrown or jerked from side to side with such rapidity, that it was impossible to distinguish his visage, and fears were entertained lest he should dislocate his neck or dash out his brains. His body partook of the same impulse, and was hurried on by like jerks, over every obstacle, — fallen trunks of trees, or, in church, over pews

---

* All these epidemics have been described and discussed by an able writer on mental disease, — Calmeil, *De la folie considérée sous le point de vue pathologique*, &c. Paris, 1845. These volumes are worthy the attention of every one interested in the study of mental phenomena.

and benches, apparently to the most imminent danger of being bruised or mangled. It was useless to attempt to hold or restrain him, and the paroxysm was permitted gradually to exhaust itself." " Sometimes the person was thrown down on the ground, when his contortions resembled those of a live fish, cast from his native element, on the land." The general character of the other exercises may be inferred from their names. As late as 1841 and 1842, a preaching epidemic broke out in Sweden, which was marked by violent convulsive movements, and involved thousands in its course.* The same phenomenon was not unfrequently witnessed in the religious movement which prevailed in Ireland in 1857 and 1858.

The epidemical character of suicide has long been recognized, and depends, no doubt, on the principle of sympathy. At the Hôtel des Invalids, in Paris, a few years since, a soldier was found, one day, dead by hanging, and within a short time twelve others hanged themselves to the same post. When the post was removed, this strange epidemic ceased. But a volume would scarcely contain the accounts of epidemic suicide that might be gathered from authentic sources. The propensity to homicide

* S. Hanbury Smith, in *Ohio Medical & Surgical Journal*, July, 1850.

is often, unquestionably, propagated in this way. In Paris, some thirty years ago, a young woman murdered her neighbor's child. The extraordinary circumstances attending the act, and the vivid discussion which it provoked among medical men, gave it an unusual degree of publicity and awakened an unusual interest in the public mind. At a session of the Academy of Medicine, Esquirol stated that, within two months after this event, there came to his knowledge six instances of attempted homicide, among persons previously correct and beyond suspicion, — led to it, according to their own statement, by reading or hearing the details of this case. Several other members, on the same occasion, bore similar testimony touching the effect of that example. This is not an insulated fact. It happened to have been observed by men who understood its full significance, and therein alone was it peculiar or exceptional.

Mania in its ordinary form never prevails epidemically, but cases not unfrequently occur in the production of which the most efficient agency is the propensity to imitation. In persons overcharged with nervous sensibility, and especially those who have inherited tendencies to mental disease, this propensity is very liable to be aroused by intimate intercourse with the insane. Many curious examples may be found in the accounts that have come down to us of demoniacal possession — that strange delusion which has furnished so many a sad and horrible chapter to the history of the race. In the early part of the seventeenth century, it made its appearance in a convent of Ursuline nuns at Loudon, France. As most of them belonged to noble families, and were highly cultivated and accomplished, they received the unstinted attentions of the clergy, many of whom were sent by the ecclesiastical authorities to endeavor, by means of all the weapons of spiritual warfare, to expel the demons from the persons and precincts of the afflicted sisterhood. Three of these exorcising priests, fathers Lactantius, Surin, and Tranquil, became possessed by the very demons they tried to cast out, the first and the last dying raving maniacs, while the other, after several paroxyms, finally recovered. The fiends which left father Tranquil in his last moments passed directly into father Lucas, who was at the bedside of the dying priest. Another scene in this Loudon tragedy furnishes additional illustration of the doctrine. Among those who were accused by these nuns of contributing to their sufferings by demoniacal means, was Urban Grandier, a priest in the village, distinguished by his mental accomplishments, by the grace of his manners and the comeliness of his person, and by some passages of gallantry somewhat at variance with modern ideas of priestly propriety. For several months their accusations were scarcely heeded, but they were artfully directed from the first by those who had good reason to hate him; and when ready to fail, they contrived to secure the all-powerful aid of Cardinal Richelieu, of whom Grandier had made a mortal enemy by means of some satirical verses. Ecclesiastical suspicion was finally roused, and judicial proceedings were ordered; but at a time when courts were creatures of the Church or State, the result could easily be foreseen. Neither his sacred office, nor his prominent position in society, nor all the graces of his mind or person, could save him from the stake; and we almost forget his vices in view of the propriety and steadiness which he displayed through every scene of his persecution, the calm but resolute assertion of his innocence, and especially the heroic — I had almost said Christian — firmness with which he encountered the final torture. Father Lactantius, who took an active part in the prosecution of Grandier, died thirty days after his victim, " in a state of fury and despair." Mannouri, the surgeon who testified that he found the devil's marks on Grandier's body, saw the ghost of the defunct priest constantly near him, until, at last, the perception became so vivid, that, on one occasion, he dropped to the ground in the excess of his terror, and died shortly after, with the dreadful image before him. Chauvet, a civil officer who bore some part in the trial, but was no believer in Grandier's guilt, was accused by one of the possessed, and, in consequence, fell into state of intense melancholy from which he never recovered.*

In the witchcraft delusion of New England, towards the close of the seventeenth century, many of the persons accused confessed that they were guilty, and described circumstantially their meetings, their intercourse with Satan, and all the performances of the Witch-Sabbath. They were, unquestionably, sincere in their confessions. Born and bred as they were in an age of superstition, believing in the personality of the devil and in his visible presence among men, ready for any wonderful tale respecting his doings, and familiarized, in this manner, with images of diabolical agency, it was but a single and an easy step to conceive — made more easy under the morbid excitement which the circumstances of a public trial were so well cal-culated to produce — that they themselves had

* Calmeil, *De la folie*, &c., ii. 54. See Trial of Urban Grandier, in *Causes celebres*, t. ii. 350, 1735.

been actual participants in the wondrous rites they had heard so vividly described. The idea once proclaimed, spread from one to another simply by force of contact.

The lesson inculcated by the facts here related should be faithfully studied and applied. Let all bear in mind that, by the very constitution of the nervous system, they are more or less disposed to sympathize in any moral, intellectual, or physical movements that may strongly arrest their attention. No one can safely consider himself as exempt from the operation of the principle in question. They who are most confident of their power of resistance, often furnish the most striking illustrations of its irresistible influence. It is incumbent on all, therefore, who know these facts, so to regulate their walk and conversation, as to expose themselves to no unnecessary danger. Intimate association with persons affected with nervous infirmities, such as chorea, hysteria, epilepsy, insanity, should be avoided by all who are endowed with a peculiarly susceptible nervous organization, whether strongly predisposed to nervous disease, or only vividly impressed by the sight of suffering and agitation. Not one of the least evils incident to insanity is, that the poor sufferer cannot receive the ministry of near relatives, without endangering the mental integ-

rity of those who offer them ; and the common
practice of removing the insane from their
own homes is required, not more for their own
welfare than the safety of those immediately
around them. Parents and teachers should
never forget that this proneness to imitate physical suffering is particularly strong in the young.
A single case of chorea or hysteria may be followed by a dozen others in the same school ;
and minor infirmities, like stuttering, and little
singularities of any kind, are imitated unconsciously, while the attention is alive, and the
organs are flexible and readily yield to every
impression.

There is a remarkable phasis of this affection
not unfrequently witnessed among persons possessing unhealthy mental tendencies, which deserves to be considered in this connection. I
refer to a morbid craving for that sympathy and
the consequent attentions, that are usually bestowed upon the sick and suffering, and which,
if not met with the proper firmness and discretion, may lead to most serious trouble. It
is confined almost, if not quite exclusively, to
young women, and accompanied by delicate
bodily health. It originates partly in a feeling
of envy, and partly in t' at propensity to imitation which is quickened and perverted by their
peculiar mental condition. They happen to

witness some case in the family or neighborhood, and the sight of the emotions and attentions to which it gives rise in others, makes a
profound impression on their minds. Thenceforth they are possessed with the desire — I say
possessed, because nothing better expresses the
fact — of achieving a position gratifying, beyond all others, to their perverted fancy. By a
process of self-deception, of which they are almost unconscious themselves, they magnify all
the little occasions of ill-health which may
really exist; conceive every unusual sensation
to be the sign of some serious affection; are
eager for drugs — the more nauseous the better — and derive satisfaction and comfort from
the paraphernalia of a sick-room. The precise
form of the ailment assumed is generally one
which they have had an opportunity of witnessing themselves, with such variations as their ingenuity may suggest. If it were a fit of hysteria, then, with a frequency which varies with
the exigences of the case, the family are thrown
into commotion by a fit of this disease, to be
again renewed as soon as the tender interest
which it excites has died away. If it were a
cold that excited some concern and led to medication and cosseting, then forthwith the house
resounds with a cough which continues proof
against the whole armory of domestic appli-

ances. No disorder, in fact, is beyond the reach
of this morbid propensity, and to such a degree
does it sometimes govern the patient, that serious injuries are self-inflicted for the purpose of
obtaining a more perfect simulation, and making
a stronger impression on the observer. Even
the power of dislocating bones at pleasure, and
of producing muscular contortions that no practicable array of force can restrain, is sometimes
exhibited in these cases. The morbid feeling at
the bottom of this affection, once fairly established, goes on gaining strength with every
day's indulgence. Suffering, at first simulated
or imagined, becomes real at last; ailments, in-
considerable in the beginning, are fostered into
strength and activity; an irritable condition of
the whole nervous system, arising, in a great degree, from the forced privations and inflictions,
becomes the source of perpetual pain or discomfort; and thus, for months, if not years,
the wretched victim of this mental perversity
remains a torment to herself and everybody
around her. Now, this ought not to be. There
is nothing mysterious in the nature of these
cases. They are well understood by those who
are conversant with mental affections, and
timely, judicious interference would always prevent their full development. Parents should
understand them, too, and be on their guard

12

against the first manifestations of the affection, in the assurance that a little wholesome discipline, with a few hints from their family physician, will be all that is necessary for their purpose.

Again, persons of striking mental peculiarities are dangerous associates to those whose minds are not happily balanced, and they are not entirely harmless to any. Their peculiarities are copied unwittingly, their ultraisms come to be regarded as not so very unreasonable, and their ridiculous fancies, and perhaps their moral shortcomings, are viewed with indulgence, if not positive favor. If blessed with large intellectual endowments, and, especially, if possessed with exaggerated ideas of their mission in life, they are apt to obtain an ascendency over others not strongly fortified by worldly experience, or a naturally healthy and symmetrical cast of mind. Their singularities of behavior are attributed by such associates to a sturdy independence of the world's opinion, and their contempt for the social institutions around them, to superior discernment and loftier aims. In spite of the repulsiveness ordinarily presented by such characters, their peculiarities strike the fancy of some who, at last, admire and imitate what, at first, was disagreeable, if not revolting. Thus, the process of assimilation goes on, step by step, until the work is entirely accomplished. On this subject nothing can be better settled than the principle, that ill-balanced minds are made still more irregular by intimate association with one another, as well as the converse principle, that nothing contributes more to keep them from farther irregularity, than the restraining influences of minds better constituted than their own. Were the importance of these views properly estimated, parents and guardians would be cautious how they selected companions and teachers whose mental qualities, though associated with good habits and principles, could not be profitably imitated by their pupils.

People of keen sensibilities and vivid conceptions cannot too carefully avoid participating in those great social movements, whether moral, political, or religious, which frequently agitate modern communities. The caution is applicable to all that class of persons whose senses are readily overpowered by the apparent magnitude of the cause which enlists their feelings, so that all others dwindle into insignificance by the side of it; whose judgment yields itself a willing captive to convictions that spring from an excited fancy, and whose emotions become so strong as to take complete possession of the man. Even they who know their danger, and determine beforehand to be moderate and prudent, are powerless before the irresistible influence which, by means of this great law of sympathy, is exerted upon them. Their prudence will avail them here as little as it would in avoiding a contagious disease to which they had needlessly exposed themselves. Most people, however, are unaware of their danger, and while they suppose themselves — quite correctly, perhaps — to be serving in a good cause, or indulging a very commendable class of feelings, they are urging every morbid tendency to the extreme limit of safety.

The law of sympathy is not controlled in its operation by the moral complexion of the thoughts and emotions which are chiefly involved. People are reluctant to believe that any subject of a commendable character, especially such as concern the highest welfare of the individual, can, even indirectly, affect the mental health. They regard it as a reflection upon Providence to suppose that what was designed to be most cheering and conservative to the soul of man, can, by any possibility, become an occasion of sorrow and disease. But the law in question conflicts with none of the analogies of nature. It is the strength and intensity of the thought or emotion, occupying the mind to the exclusion of all other thoughts and emotions, and predominating over all other interests, that produce the evil. This alone is the essential condition. It matters not whether the movement that arrests the attention is moral, political, or religious; whether it be to strike a blow for freedom or slavery; to promote the triumph of virtue or of vice; to produce contrition for sin or brazen persistence in wrong; to strengthen the arm of the law, or help the spirit of misrule; the healthy balance of the faculties is equally liable to be disturbed. Indeed, the more worthy the subject may be to excite the interest of a rational creature, and secure his most serious consideration, so much the more liable are persons of a susceptible temperament to be moved beyond the measure of a healthy excitement.

The course of our remarks leads us to consider another mental condition very intimately connected with the health of the mind. When the thoughts and emotions are deeply engrossed with a particular subject, their ordinary current is generally accelerated, and perhaps to a high degree of rapidity. To pitch the mental movements on a scale very different from that on which they usually proceed is not a healthy operation, however satisfactory or agreeable may be its immediate results. Where this often happens, the mind is liable to lose at last some portion of its native vigor, and become, it may

be, a prey to actual disorder. As a people, we
are remarkably prone to mental excitement. It
is common in almost everybody's experience,
and forms the habitual condition of many. It
would seem as if moderation, quiet, and steady
application, in the pursuits of life, were entitled
to little respect, and as if no object calculated to
awaken much interest could be followed, except
under the pressure of excitement. Occasions
are frequently occurring when large bodies of
men are moved by this spirit, and when even
the whole surface of society rolls and swells
under its potent influence. One of these occasions, for instance, is furnished quadrennially,
by the Presidential election, which enlists the
feelings of every man, if not every woman, in
the land. For days and weeks and months
together, the predominant sentiment is manifested, at home and abroad, by day and by
night, in season and out of season, by the fire-
side and in the market-place, in private inter-
views and public gatherings, in mass meetings
and evening processions, in lectures and sermons and speeches innumerable, as if the dearest
interests of the individual depended on the
result. Another prolific occasion of mental
excitement is furnished by those religious awakenings which have occurred among us with
remarkable frequency and spread to a remark-

able extent. The language just used to describe
political exeitement requires but little modifi-
cation to be equally applicable to this. The
hygienic effect upon the mind, in the two cases,
may be different; and it is not improbable, that
if the grounds of this difference were better
understood, the subject might be freely discussed
without exciting the alarm of truly religious
people.

A little examination will show us that accidental incidents may greatly modify the result
— may make all the difference between a form
of excitement not directly injurious, and one
which may pass, by easy gradations, into positive disease. The latter may be accompanied
with an utter disregard of the plainest rules for
the preservation of the bodily health. Food
may be taken irregularly, and the functions of
the stomach thus disordered; the body, imperfectly clad, perhaps, may be exposed to atmospherical changes, and thus the sympathy
between the skin and the lungs be deranged;
the hours that should be given to repose may
be surrendered to the all-absorbing topic, and
for want of the blessed influences which "tired
nature's sweet restorer" diffuses over the whole
system, animal and organic, there may occur a
morbid irritability that deepens the impression
made by every adverse incident; habits of daily

exercise and recreation, which have become essential to the physical welfare, may be entirely abandoned, and the brain no longer visited by the invigorating influences that radiate from the muscular system. Any one of these incidents may impart to the mental excitement an unhealthy character, and convert it into actual disease.

It must be considered, also, that on these occasions of prevalent excitement, those habitual exercises of the mind which are promotive of peace, cheerfulness, and serenity ; that active interest in the welfare of others which withdraws one from a too steady devotion to selfish objects; and especially those glimpses of a higher and brighter sphere above the agitations of flesh and sense, — frequent in the experience of some, and not entirely withheld from any, — all these may be completely absorbed in the thought or emotion that holds possession of the individual.

The ultimate effect of mental excitement depends very much on its character. If it grat-ifies the pleasing emotions ; if it inspires hope and joy ; if is attended with hilarity and merriment ; and, especially, if the objects in view are not too closely connected with the immediate personal welfare, — then its consequences are far less injurious than if the predominant feelings are of a depressing character, such as intense apprehensions of coming evil, an overwhelming sense of unworthiness and shortcoming, and a fear of personal danger. Strong emotions of any kind, indulged in for a considerable period, are not conducive to mental health, but I believe it is the opinion of those most conversant with the subject, that the pleasing kind are less liable to this result than those of a painful or disagreeable character.

Other qualities of the emotion besides those of pleasure or pain, may determine, in some degree, its effect on the mind. Many a person who experiences safely the joy arising from the sudden acquisition of property or the reunion of friends, or even the grief that follows calamity or death, would quail before some startling incident having in it a tinge of mystery or wonder.

Bearing in mind these facts, we may readily see why the mental health sustains so little harm, comparatively, from intense political excitement, even when intensified, as it now is, by a struggle for national existence. It seldom affects a person's habits of living. He takes his meals and exercise as regularly as ever, and with as keen a relish; his sleep is sound and his conscience quiet; his sympathies are not entirely silenced; he acknowledges the claim of his

neighbor to a helping hand; and his eye and
ear are not utterly closed to everything else
that is passing around him. The danger he
apprehends, the good he seeks, are somewhat
remote; and upon few, comparatively, of those
who mingle in political strife will the result
have any immediate personal bearings. Their
business, their social position, their domestic
affections, their fortune, all remain the same,
whether the favorite candidate succeed or fail.
The emotions which spring from the joy of
success, or the pain of failure, seldom come
from the depths of the soul, and cannot with-
stand the intrusion of other sentiments more
nearly connected with the ordinary experience.
I do not mean to convey the impression that,
in a hygienic point of view, political excitement
is entirely harmless, directly or indirectly. It is
one form or phasis of that excessive mental
activity so characteristic of our times, which
may be fairly considered as having much to do
with the present increasing prevalence of mental
disease. A more particular examination of its
effects, however, must be reserved for another
division of this inquiry.

Religious excitement, it is well known, has
the credit of producing numerous cases of mental disorder, much to the embarrassment and
uneasiness of many worthy people, who cannot

understand how so beneficent an agency as religion should ever produce such disastrous results. The evil in question must be attributed, however, not to religion, but to a certain form of excitement by which it is frequently, though not necessarily accompanied. The fact that insanity is often produced in this way cannot fairly be denied; and it is the part of true religion as well as true philosophy, to recognize the evil, and provide, if possible, a suitable remedy. Passionate declamation, and charges of infidelity against the conscientious observer, convince no one who is anxious to know the truth of the matter. They only raise the suspicion that the cause is weak which can show no better support than these.

To explain the extraordinary prevalence and intensity of this emotion at certain seasons, — its secondary causes, so to speak, to distinguish them from the spiritual agency supposed to be always present, — we have only to consider the impressions and influences to which our people have been generally subjected. In this country, no subject, probably, occupies the attention of so large a number of persons, with so high a degree of interest, as religion, in some of its forms and developments. At first sight, this may seem incompatible with the existing amount of depravity, but it will be obvious, on

a little reflection, that both facts may be strictly
true. Religious institutions are so widely
diffused and respected, that comparatively few
can pass through their childhood without receiving impressions that may never be effaced.
Doctrines are received, passively, perhaps, but
with none the less confidence in their truth;
while even the knotty points of controversial
divinity are discussed, not exclusively by scholars and critics. Even those who forget the
requirements of religion and are careless of its
obligations, cherish in their inmost heart a certain regard for its sanctions, and pay to it a
kind of involuntary homage. It is not strange,
therefore, that, in seasons of unusual interest in
the subject, the religious sentiment, however
dormant, should be revived and quickened in
multitudes, and the most indifferent reminded
that there are higher objects within our reach
than this life can furnish.

These views are strikingly confirmed by the
character of the delusions that agitate the minds
of the insane. In the New England hospitals
— and I particularize them, merely because I
am better acquainted with them than with any
others — the delusions of a considerable proportion of the patients are of a religious complexion; and it must be borne in mind, that in this
description of cases are many never supposed to

have a religious origin. I presume there may
be found in those institutions, at any time, those
who imagine they have sinned away the day
of grace, or committed the unpardonable sin,
or are doomed to eternal perdition. They may
not have been distinguished for remarkable
deficiency, or remarkable sensitiveness. They
may not have been dwelling upon religious subjects in an unusual manner, just previous to the
attack. It would seem as if, at the moment the
mind had lost its power of controlling the
thoughts, a host of religious impressions, long
latent, perhaps, but never entirely effaced, were
suddenly revived with that kind of vividness
which only disease can impart; and instead of
serving merely as serious admonitions to duty,
they prove a whip of scorpions, lacerating and
torturing to the utmost limit of endurance.
Now it must be considered that the delusions
of the insane do not spring out of the ground,
but originate, more or less remotely in their own
mental experience; and this is the reason why
the delusions of our patients are so frequently
of a religious character.

There is another reason why religious excitement, beyond all other forms of excitement,
should derange the healthy balance of the mental
faculties, and that is the superior magnitude of
the interests with which it is concerned. They

are no holiday matter which one may attend to or neglect without materially affecting his immediate welfare. They involve nothing less than his future destiny, and are well calculated, if anything is, to produce serious thought, if not overwhelming emotion. They also include an element of personal danger, sufficient to excite apprehensions that seldom accompany the gloomiest forebodings of those, for instance, who are strongly exercised by political grievances. A sense of responsibility, quickened by the consciousness of past deficiencies and neglected opportunities, also helps to sharpen sensibilities already alive and glowing with excitement.

If these views are correct, there can be no question as to their practical application in the conduct and business of men. Although moderation, equanimity, and prudence are inculcated, in general terms, both by philosophy and hygiene, yet the majority of mankind require a more stringent rule of action; and in this case, they will find it in the immediate danger that accompanies excessive indulgence in many, if not all, the forms of mental excitement. Excesses of this kind, as well as of many others, may be followed, in most cases, by no appreciable amount of harm; but it must be recollected that hygienic rules are made, not so much for the sound and strong, as for those whose stamina are impaired, and who thereby have become extremely susceptible to every adverse influence around them. In every throng which is moved by some popular excitement may be found those who have inherited a disposition to mental disease, which needs only some occasion of this kind to be actually developed; those whose nervous system is so irritable that any departure from the ordinary routine of thought and emotion produces a degree of agitation ever liable to pass beyond the limit of safety; those whose sympathies, uncontrolled by the restraints of reason and propriety, are irresistibly impelled to imitate every extravagance they witness; those whose perceptions of right and wrong, of the true and the false, are always accompanied by a feverish glow of emotion, which, instead of strengthening and elevating, only frets and chafes the spirit. These are the persons who cannot engage in scenes of excitement without imminent danger of losing the nice adjustment of their faculties and becoming the subjects of actual disease. I do not suppose that excite-ment can be banished from every sphere of human activity, or that such a result would be desirable, if it could. It has its uses, and within certain limits it furnishes indispensable aid in realizing the purposes and aspirations of men.

But the duty of avoiding it is no less imperative on some persons than that of avoiding indigestible food on the part of the feeble and dyspeptic. To say that all may safely indulge in excitement, because it is a natural condition of the constitution which God has given us, is no better logic than it would be to contend that strong food must be salutary under all circumstances, because it is the gift of God. Let those, too, whose position enables them to control and direct the course of popular excitement, remember that they are under a fearful responsibility for the manner in which they exert their power. Their cause may be good, the object desirable, but they are none the less bound to be careful how they seek to accomplish it by a system of means that may involve the ruin of multitudes.

The voice of admonition too often falls on unwilling ears, for people are slow to believe that exercises which are highly meritorious, because leading to a good result, and prompted, perhaps, by divine influence, can, by any possibility, be dangerous to the mental health. Indeed, it seems to them little short of impiety to suppose it. Let them remember that they are yet in the flesh; that no pursuit or exercise, however commendable, can be successfully followed by a system of means not in accordance with the laws of the animal economy. They may be sure that these will not be suspended to enable them to accomplish a desirable end ; and they may be also sure that divine influences are always in harmony with those natural laws which have proceeded from the same beneficent source. Those who are sincerely desirous of guarding against the development of morbid tendencies, should carefully avoid all scenes of religious excitement, and indulge their religious emotions in quiet and by ordinary methods, always allowing other emotions and other duties their rightful share of attention. Regulated in this manner, the religious sentiment will be to them, not only a source of spiritual comfort, but a power more efficient, it may be, than any other, for maintaining the healthy balance of the faculties, and keeping in abeyance the hereditary proclivities to disease.

Let me not be misunderstood. God forbid that I should wish to undervalue the benefits of true religion. Of all the influences exerted upon the mind, none are more conservative of its health and vigor than that of the great truths of Christianity, clearly discerned, and properly applied to the life. They, and they alone, sometimes, are capable of keeping it sure and steadfast under the trials that assail it, exalting and strengthening while they preserve. And yet among the countless varieties of the mental

13

constitution, it is not strange that some should
want that elasticity which enables it to resist
the shock of unusual commotions, as well as
the power of converting momentous truths into
materials of enduring life and health. It is idle
to question so obvious a fact.

To those who demand particular facts on
this subject, I would submit the following statement respecting a class of cases deplorably
familiar to those who have charge of hospitals
devoted to the care of the insane. " The number of instances in which insanity is stated to
have originated in religious excitement has been
very considerable; but in seven only could I
satisfy myself after the most careful and candid
examination, that such was really the case. In
these, the patients' relatives had no doubt whatever as to the origin of their attack, and each
of them after recovery — for they all recovered
— most unhesitatingly corroborated that opinion. Four of them were persons of strong religious convictions before the commencement
of the Revival Movement; and I ascertained
that the other three had led regular and exem-
plary lives for some years previous to their illness. It is a common impression — and, as far
as my limited experience goes, an erroneous
one — that, in such cases, the terrors of hell and
a future judgment held up to the excited im-

aginaton act immediately in disturbing the mental equilibrium. The individuals alluded to above, on the contrary, either had, or believed they had, 'found peace'; and it was the over-whelming excitement and joy attendant on this belief that produced insanity. The mind, con-stantly occupied with one subject, neglect of regular hours, want of sleep, late and early at-tendance on prayer-meetings, foolish attempts to teach others, (a vocation for which they were ill adapted,) — in fact, a direct contravention of the laws of mental and physical health, com-bined to produce their natural result — mental disease. One gentleman succumbed to the anxiety and distress occasioned by unsuccessful attempts to address an audience. Another was so overjoyed by his conversion that he scarcely ate or slept for a week; and his joy culminated in an attack of most violent mania. A man who became affected by powerful emotional disturbance was considered by those who had seen such cases in Ireland to be a genuine ex-ample of 'striking down,' and he was treated accordingly, until his 'physical manifestations,' became of too turbulent a character to be con-trolled out of an asylum." *

In the course of that great awakening which

* DR. HOWDEN, in *Report of Lunatic Asylum of Montrose,* Scotland, for 1860.

occurred in this country in 1857 and 1858, the
following case came under my own observation.
A worthy couple, in one of our principal cities,
had pursued the even tenor of their way, until
they had arrived at the period of middle life.
They were correct in their life and conversation,
and their religious observances, like those of
many others, consisted in going to church on
Sundays. On this occasion, seeing their friends
and neighbors frequenting the meetings, they,
too, solely in the spirit of imitation, concluded
to go. They immediately became absorbed in
the subjects presented to their attention, to the
exclusion of every other consideration. On the
third or fourth day it was obvious they were
losing their reason, and within a week from the
time when they began to attend the meetings,
they were both raving maniacs, and such they
died, one, in the course of a few days, the other
in the fourth week. One of them had inherited
a predisposition to mental disease, though it
had never before made its appearance; but, of
the other, in this respect, I knew nothing.

The case-books of every hospital for the insane abound with cases illustrating the same
doctrine. And the lesson which such facts
teach is, not that religious awakenings are un-
mitigated evils, because there is abundant evidence to the contrary, but that they should be

carefully shunned by all who have any predisposition to mental disease.

The connection between mind and body is
regulated by laws that cannot be disregarded
without risk of serious detriment to both. That
the bodily organs may be directly affected by
mental impressions is a matter of daily observation, and the medical man who is thoroughly
acquainted with the resources of his art, will
resort to them with no less confidence in their
efficacy, than in that of drugs and plasters. In
a large proportion of cases, they may be made,
if dexterously managed, far more conducive to
the restoration of health, than any amount of
the latter. In this way, I account for most of
the salutary effect of journeys and voyages and
watering-places; and even famous methods of
cure are oftener indebted for their success to the
hopeful state of mind they excite than to any
direct action upon the suffering organ. In accordance with a similar law, the depressing
passions impair the vital energies and invite the
approaches of disease. It is an undoubted fact
that the prevalence of cholera, not to mention other epidemics, has always been greatly
promoted by the fear of an attack. Nor can it
be doubted that sporadic diseases have occasionally been communicated in the same way.
In 1824, a man died in Guy's Hospital, London,

with all the symptoms of hydrophobia, which
he began to manifest immediately after reading
a newspaper account of a case of this disease.

The hygienic condition of the mind is not less
influenced by the character of its passions and
emotions, its habitual temper and disposition.
In a man of cheerful spirit and hopeful views
of life, the mental health is less likely to be impaired, other things being equal, than in one
who is easily depressed by trial, and fond of
looking upon the dark side of things. Let this
frame of mind become firmly established, and
we shall have taken the first step in the path
which leads to mental disease ; for many of the
forms of insanity seem to be but exaggerations
of moral qualities, which, primarily, were simply
uncomfortable or disagreeable. A cross and
fretful temper is also prejudicial to the mental
health, because it prevents the mind from bearing up under the trials of life with proper
serenity, and by long indulgence becomes transformed, very often, into actual disease. The
advice of Feuchtersleben is worthy of all acceptation, whether we adopt his theory or not.
" When a man has had the misfortune to be
born ill-humored, he should not, as most do,
deceive himself; he should rather regard himself as laboring under disease, and employ every
means in his power to get rid of the affliction."

In the education of the young, the discipline of
the passions is of the highest importance, in a
hygienic point of view.   A child who is habitually peevish and fretful, who manifests frequent paroxysms of anger and chafes under the
lightest restrictions, will require a large endowment of some restraining grace, to escape the
formation of mental habits as uncontrollable
as they are odious.   When we consider how
large a portion of the time children are in the
care of servants possessing little culture or principle, and who would naturally seek to maintain their control by playing on the feelings of
their charge, it is not wonderful that insanity
should be one of those diseases, the increase of
which seems to be favored by the progress of
civilization.   When a child is frightened to
death by some raw-head-and-bloody-bones story
of its nurse, the cause, the effect, the mode of
operation, are obvious to the dullest observer,
but when the impression is lighter, though not
readily erased, and the final result more remote,
we fail to observe the intermediate steps, and
attribute to a mysterious dispensation of Providence what is chiefly the effect of bad domestic
training.

Among the mental exercises and conditions
under the control of the individual, few, probably, have a greater effect on the vigor of the

mind than habit. In general terms this is universally acknowledged, and the old adage, that
habit is second nature, equally expresses the
popular and the philosophical belief. In regard
to the bodily organs, there has been no hesitation in recognizing and turning to practical account this power of habit. We easily teach
the muscles to execute with the utmost rapidity
a complicated series of motions, with the least
possible exercise of the will. The lungs, the
stomach, the muscles, we invigorate by appropriate habits, which, however difficult and disagreeable at first, become at last easy and
pleasing. The mind is no less under the power
of habit than the body. Its power of continuous and vigorous thought, as well as its fondness for dreams and reveries; its aspirations for
the good and the true, and its proclivities for
the mean and the sordid; its taste for the grand
and the beautiful, and its affinities for the low
and the grovelling, may, each and all, be confirmed and developed by the force of habit.

By habits of mind I mean such mental exercises as we are accustomed to perform with some
degree of regularity, — and, thus defined, I do
not hesitate to say that they produce the same
promptitude and facility of execution which
follow the frequent repetition of bodily movements. It seems to be a law of our mental

constitution, somewhat analogous to that law of periodicity which is observed in the actions of the nervous system, that emotions, propensities, and processes of thought, once distinctly manifested, tend to repeat themselves, automatically, as it were. This law is curiously illustrated in the latter stages of protracted mental disease, where all active manifestations of mind have long since disappeared. These wrecks of humanity, incapable of originating the simplest process of thought, may be observed executing a complicated piece of music with as much correctness as in their best days, or playing at checkers or cards with but little diminution of their accustomed skill. Their attention needs only to be directed to a familiar point, and the necessary mental movements succeed one another by some mysterious process of association. The operation of the law is visible, even in those exercises which seem to require some effort of thought. Sentence will follow after sentence, disjointed and incongruous, perhaps, but not wanting in a certain semblance of logic, or eloquence, or wisdom.

The working of the mind is governed by the same laws in health as in disease, and no one much accustomed to observe it in himself or others, can have failed to witness the influence of habit even in those exercises which seem most independent of it. In speaking and writing, for instance, the thoughts follow one another, automatically, in a great degree, without any conscious effort of the thinking power. A man sits down at his table, with only the most imperfect conception of what he shall write, but thought after thought leaps forth, clothed in appropriate words, and the result is something which instructs and delights the world. A public speaker rises in his place, with only some general outline of what he intends to say, but the tongue is directed by an unceasing force, the right thing is said in the right place, and not only do arguments and images arise, almost unbidden, but while uttering the beginning of a sentence, the mind looks forward and conceives and arranges the next. Now, without pretending to furnish a complete explanation of these mental processes, it can hardly be questioned that this rapidity of movement is in a great degree one of the results of habit. Therefore, to derive the utmost amount of benefit from this law of our nature, care should be taken that our mental habits be rightly ordered. If they are regular and systematic, suited to the taste and abilities, and characterized by some activity and effort, they will impart to the exercises of the mind that ease and readiness of performance in which their efficiency so much consists. If, on the other hand, they are desultory and fitful, governed only by whim or caprice, and involving only the lower faculties, they make none of those permanent furrows, if I may use the figure, which guide and facilitate the courses of thought.

The force of habit is no less powerful in perpetuating moral and intellectual peculiarities, and the fact should always be borne in mind by those who are entrusted with the care of the young. Upon them it may depend, whether an objectionable trait of character shall be eradicated by timely attention, or firmly established and thus become, at last, a prolific source of unhappiness, if not overt disease. The manner in which the latter result is brought about is well described in the following paragraph: " Some are led to begin this course of error by distinct and well-marked tastes for it. In others, a feeling is accidentally excited; it may be very slight at first, but by repetition it gains strength, and ultimately becomes powerful. This is remarkably manifested in the caprices and perversities. The mind capriciously determines to be pleased with a small point, and through this sees all the rest. This prepossession compels the perceptive faculties to present the acceptable trait first to the mind, and put it in good humor to see those associated with it,

and then it looks upon them, at last, with toleration. By repetition, the toleration becomes
satisfaction, and approbation follows after. At
last, the whole mind is brought under the power
of the caprice ; then opinions are formed, and a
course of conduct pursued, from which the reason at first would have shrunk ; but, being dis-
armed and made the servant of passion or
caprice, it goes to strengthen the error and over-
throw the judgment." *

Youth, undoubtedly, is the most proper period
for the formation of good habits of mind, and
in the education of the young this great end
should never be overlooked. The ability to do
a thing does not always insure its performance,
and unless it can be done without much effort,
and with a measure of satisfaction, it will
scarcely be done at all. Nobody supposes that
a musical performer, however correct his ear,
would derive any pleasure from the exercise,
were he always obliged, like a beginner, to
direct every movement of his fingers by a special, deliberate act of the will. And yet, as education is commonly managed, it seems to be
supposed that certain attainments in knowledge,
and the recognition of certain moral distinctions, comprise all that we need. To make

* Dr. EDWARD JARVIS, in Barnard's *American Journal of Education*, March, 1858, p. 602.

these things a part of ourselves by reducing them to practice ; to make them easy and familiar by habit, and thus alone to make them available for any good purpose, is not generally recognized as a legitimate result of education. And yet no one doubts that the great results of life are determined not so much by what men know, as by the facility and discretion with which they use that knowledge. The little learning of some men proves infinitely more serviceable in the business of life, than the abundant knowledge of others. Even the plainest lesson of morality and religion may bear no fruit unless incorporated into the habits of the individual. To say, be upright, be benevolent, be self-denying, will be of no more avail in forming the moral character, than an attempt to relieve the bodily wants by saying, be ye clothed, or be ye fed.

The mental efficiency of most men is more or less impaired by improper habits of mental occupation. They go through life with a large amount of latent power undeveloped, and utterly unable to concentrate their energies on any particular point. To accomplish the most with a given amount of original endowment is a result that can come only from a course of suitable discipline ; and many a man whose mind has grown up at hap-hazard, under the impulses of the moment, without method or management; active to-day and idle to-morrow; at one time, exploring a subject with commendable zeal and diligence, and at another resigning himself to idle reveries or superficial study, fails to make good the promise of his early days. In whatever situation a person of any intellectual tastes may be placed, the health and vigor of his mind may be materially increased by some system in its use and exercise. In regard to the special pursuits whereby men obtain their living, I need not speak in this relation; but every man has, or ought to have, his hours of leisure, and the manner in which these are spent will determine, in a great degree, his happiness and efficiency. From a feeling of weariness, real or imaginary, or, it may be, from downright indolence, many eschew every description of mental exercise at those times, but such as conduce to the entertainment of the hour. Unquestionably there are conditions of mind when a novel or a play will furnish it with more salutary exercise, than studies requiring more thought and closer application. They serve then the purpose of recreation, and the mind is enabled to resume its customary work, refreshed and invigorated. Like all indulgences which are salutary enough when temperately used, this is liable to become habitual, and thus indispose a man to any mental

employments requiring activity and perseverance.

Persons whose habitual employment requires
considerable mental activity during several hours
of the day, will best obtain the recreation they
need by some kind of mental exercise which,
without being fatiguing, requires just enough of
effort to impart a degree of interest and satisfaction to the result. They need, not so much absolute quietude, as a change of subject which
calls into action a different order of faculties
from those which have already been fatigued.
A man's special pursuits are generally a matter
of toil and taskwork, from which he gladly
turns to something that appeals to his taste or
fancy rather than to his needs. True, it may
still be the higher faculties that are thus em-
ployed, but instead of the same daily routine,
the employment is constantly suggesting new
thoughts and new scenes, and being pursued at
will, without restriction or limitation, the interest is steadily maintained. It is well to have
some pet employment for one's leisure hours,
with sufficient dignity to redeem it from the
charge of frivolity and add a zest to the gratification it affords. The merchant who retires to
his farm, and dismisses all thought of traffic
while pruning his trees or discussing the qualities of his stock; the lawyer or doctor who re-

lieves his professional toils by investigating some favorite subject remote from the ordinary sphere of his labors ; the merchant's clerk, who, when the work of the day is finished, gladly turns to his book of history or biography ; the mechanic or farmer who always finds an opportunity for learning the events of the time, or adding, in some way, to his stock of ideas, obtain a more durable gratification, and do more to repair the wear and tear produced by their more arduous occupations, than they would by devouring heaps of novels, or resorting to scenes of amusement.

These views cannot be too strongly urged upon our countrymen, with whom unceasing toil is not so much a matter of necessity as it is among less favored nations, and who are much inclined to seek for recreation in idleness or frivolous amusement.

In another respect, the mental habits of our people are detrimental to the health and vigor of the mind. With all our ambition and energy, we need, above all things, more steadiness in our pursuits, and a more diligent application. With a set task before us, on which some special object is depending, no people can accomplish more ; but without such an object in view, especially without the stimulus of necessity, no people are more prone to spend their time in doing nothing, or what amounts to scarcely anything. How many start in life under the impression that the great objects of worldly success are to be obtained, not so much by patient and persevering industry, as by some happy stroke of fortune. The slow rewards of diligence and painstaking prudence have no charms for men whose eyes are fixed on the more rapid and brilliant results of adroit management, or bold speculation, or hazardous adventure. So long as the latter evade our grasp, we imagine that we have mistaken our calling, that better fortune is in store for us, did we but know where to seek it, and forthwith we look about for some opportunity to change. Thus we become unstable and unsteady in our ways; repeated disappointment and vexation destroy the healthy elasticity of the mind, and the idleness that necessarily follows a frequent change of pursuit contributes nothing to its strength. The old adage, that the devil is always at the elbow of an idle man, is almost literally true in this relation. The unoccupied mind is the sport of every whim and impulse, driven about by vague desires and impracticable schemes, and a prey to any morbid emotion or extravagant idea that in the chapter of accidents may turn up. At this point its downward progress becomes more rapid, until it ends in hopeless

14

ennui or overt insanity. I have no hesitation, therefore, in saying that of all the means for preserving the health, there is nothing more sure, or better suited to a greater variety of persons, than habits of regular and systematic mental occupation of some dignity and worth.

In this proposition I would embrace all those kinds of employment which pass under the general name of business, and which, little as we are sometimes disposed to recognize the fact, bears the same relation to the health of the mind, that food, exercise, &c., do to the health of the body. Work is the condition of our being, as active and progressive creatures; and if performed with due regard to the constitution of the individual and the nature of the employment, it will do more, probably, than any other single agency, to maintain the native energies, both of body and mind. No advantages of fortune or of station can place us entirely beyond its necessity, and no one whose life is spent in a round of frivolous pursuits, has a right to reckon upon that vigor and elasticity of mind which will sustain it under the trials of adversity, or the morbid influences that may flow from other parts of the system. Few of us, I imagine, are fully aware how much we owe on this score, to those daily recurring pursuits which fix our thoughts and task our energies. The doctor who begins his tour of duty in the early hours of morning, and scarcely ends it with the shades of evening; the lawyer who, day after day, renews his conflicts at the bar, or deliberations in chambers; the merchant who hurries from the breakfast-table to the counting-room, to rejoice or to chafe over the account of sales and purchases which the morning's mail has laid on his desk; the school-master, the bank-clerk, the shopkeeper, and all the host of employés who are expected to be at their posts at the striking of the clock; the farmer and the mechanic, whose toil is longer, if not more harassing, — let them all consider that in their several allotments of labor are essential conditions of their health and happiness. Employment which is steadily pursued as a part of the established routine of life, and felt to be, in some degree, a matter of necessity, has an effect on the mind far more salutary than that which depends on the impulse of the moment, and is determined by no sense of necessity nor force of habit. There can be no question that the very regularity with which the stated task returns is congenial to the mental constitution, answering, perhaps, to that law of periodicity by which the actions of the nervous system are greatly controlled. The long-settled habit of pursuing some specific employment cannot be

discontinued without serious danger to the
mind, which, deprived of the customary object
of its thoughts and cares, becomes a prey to
ennui, if nothing worse. The story of the tal-
low-chandler, who, on retiring from business,
retained the privilege of being present on dip-
ping days, may raise a smile, but it illustrates
an important truth. In England, where habits
are more firmly fixed than with us, the liability
of old persons to become insane after withdraw-
ing from their customary pursuits, is distinctly
noticed by some of her best writers on the disease. The remarks on this point of an English
writer who, with remarkable skill, has treated of
those mental peculiarities which are compatible with unquestionable sanity, though indicative, certainly, of abnormal mental action, deserve to be pondered well by all to whom they
can possibly be applied: "A man accustomed
to business, and possessed of an active mind,
and who has lived amid the excitements of a
large city and a numerous acquaintance, if suddenly removed from such a kind of life to a
country house, or to a country town, finds that
by far the worst part of the change consists in
the removal of an excitement, the effects of
which were not fully known to him before.
Withdrawn in a great degree from external objects, the attention becomes strongly and almost

continually directed inwards; a state which has
sometimes been considered as affording opportunity for a review of past conduct, and the formation of good resolutions, but in which, in reality, the mind, if not wholly occupied about the
faults of others, generally dwells on its own
movements and its own feelings, until the importance of both becomes exceedingly exaggerated. This state proves to many quite unfavorable to the quiet pursuit of science or literature; the imagination has an irregular exercise;
and indolence produces self-reproach and despondency. A suspicion begins to be felt that
the mind has not only lost its habits of activity,
but also its power to undertake any employment demanding perseverance. The want of
external excitement comes at last to be made
up for by various sources of mental agitation,
which are only rendered important by continuance or frequent succession; and it is found
with surprise, that the facility once possessed of
profiting by short intervals of leisure is sup-
planted by an inability to do anything well
when there is nothing to be done. In such a
situation, the declension of the mind may be
observed, from activity to indolence, and from
indolence to that state of apathy which is very
little removed from a state of sleep. Even a
devotion to the common pleasures of sense is

better than such a state of absolute indifference;
for if even these give no kind of pleasure, whilst
all higher pursuits are neglected, there is danger
lest a man become of the same opinion as Dr.
Darwin's patient, ' that all which life affords is a
ride out in the morning, and a warm parlor and
a pack of cards in the afternoon '; and like him,
finding these pleasures not inexhaustible, should
shoot himself because he has nothing better to
do."

" Even amidst the excitement of the capital,
the want of those continual motives to industry
which arise from a profession, or from some regular pursuit in life, or from the necessity of
making some provision for others, or from any
of those privations and difficulties of which the
operation is always beneficial, though seldom
duly appreciated, is most fatal to mental ease.
A condition which most men would choose, because apparently including every blessing of nature and fortune, has been known to become
tormenting and intolerable. The possession of
wealth and rank, a liberal education, great liter
ary acquirements, many accomplishments, correctness of life, elegance of manners, and extraordinary powers of conversation, together
with the frequent enjoyment of a society in
which all these particulars are fully estimated,
present a combination of advantages which

very few possess, and to which none can be indifferent: if anything could promise worldly
happiness, such a combination of natural and
acquired endowments would seem to do so.
They were never, perhaps, more happily united
than in the instance of Mr. Topham Beauclerk,
the friend and frequent companion of Johnson,
by whom, as indeed by all the great men of a
time in which great men abounded, he was not
only admired but beloved. Yet we are told
that the activity or the restlessness of his mind
required something more; and that, sometimes
unsatisfactorily engaged in desultory studies,
and sometimes in dissipation, and sometimes in
play, he was too often a martyr to misanthropy,
and querulousness, and ennui. At such times,
it cannot be doubted that there was an approach to disease of mind." *

In this connection it is proper to refer to a
feature of this our modern life, evincing a deplorable disregard of this law of our mental
constitution. I mean the absence of stated,
useful employment on the part of the female
members of families in easy circumstances.
The little accomplishments of needle-work, so
generally diffused, can hardly be dignified with
the name of work, for though they give the appearance of occupation, they furnish no exercise

* Conolly, J. *Indications of Insanity*, p. 182.

to body or mind, and might be entirely dispensed with without detriment to anybody. I would not censure any for abstaining from employments better left to those who need the compensation they afford. But it is a poor view of woman's duties and capacities, that confines her to a little busy idleness, because the chances of fortune have placed her beyond the necessity of earning her living; and they must have but a narrow view of the exigencies of social life who believe that any woman of tolerable health and strength may not find abundant opportunities of that kind of work which affords no other recompense than the consciousness of doing good, and therefore to be done, if done at all, by those who can dispense with every other compensation. A life of idleness and luxurious ease can be no more honorable to one sex than to the other, and we know very well, that in a man, it creates no claims upon the respect and confidence of the community. The time is coming, it is to be hoped, when every right-minded, true-hearted woman will feel that she is designed for something better than a mere butterfly existence consisting chiefly of dress, crochet, novels, and parties, and determine to devote that leisure which she owes to the allotments of a kind Providence, to those benevolent ministrations which her nature renders her so well-fitted to perform. That the work in question has been actually begun, that many a benevolent enterprise has been conceived and carried forward by this class of persons, is confirmatory evidence that the views here advanced are sound, practicable, and adapted to the wants of the time. But this kind of work is never finished, and the utmost possible influx of laborers would be scarcely sufficient for the harvest. Nothing but the practical application of these remarks can save many a mind, liberally and beautifully endowed, from that series of mental ills which begins with habitual vacuity and ends with actual insanity. True, this is not the invariable result, thanks to a good constitution and the benevolent appliances of nature; but let a little ill-health, or an hereditary taint, or a great affliction, throw its weight into the scale, and then it may be reasonably expected.

Important as stated employment unquestionably is, to the mental health, amusement or recreation is scarcely less so. Few persons, whatever their mental character or temperament, can safely dispense with them altogether. At some time or other, in some shape or other, they would exert a salutary influence upon all who suffer the wear and tear of labor whether of body or mind. Even the most commanding intellects sometimes seek the recreation which

their exhausting labors make necessary, in forms
of amusement which, to those who feel the
necessity less, seem to be frivolous and puerile.
For this purpose, Bayle was not ashamed of
witnessing the performances of Punch and Judy.
William Pinkney was accustomed to unbend
over the flimsiest productions of the Minerva
Press, and Daniel Webster was in the habit of
repairing to the sea-shore, to recruit his exhausted energies by fishing from his boat. True,
most persons of this class find sufficient recreation in some form of mental activity, less than
is required by their stated employments, and
many others of somewhat smaller intellect and
humbler calling might profitably do the same
in some degree. But it can hardly be doubted
that, to all classes whose habitual pursuits require more head than hand, a judicious resort
to amusements would be attended with the happiest effects. Endowed, as we are, with the
faculty of being amused, — of deriving gratification from things that only excite our mirth, — it
seems to be a reflection on the Author of our
being, to regard amusements as something to
be carefully shunned, rather than sought and
enjoyed. Their legitimate effect, when properly
managed, is yet to be experienced among us,
because they have hitherto been too much de-
based by associations that do not rightfully

belong to them. In order that they may invigorate rather than enervate the mind, they should be used with due moderation, and never as a means of fostering merely nervous excitement; they should appeal to none of the lower sentiments or propensities; they should stimulate no passion, nor contribute, in any way, to disturb the bodily health.

To that larger class in every community, whose life is one of severe toil and harassing cares, amusements constitute almost the only practicable means for repairing the constant waste of the nervous energy. If, in this country, it is more disposed to mental disease than the corresponding classes of the Old World, it may be accounted for, in some degree, by the fact that the latter devote a much larger portion of their leisure to social intercourse and festive enjoyments. Among the most imperative of our social wants is a better supply of cheap and innocent amusements adapted to the national tastes and customs. Especially is this want felt by the female sex, in the humbler walks of life, whose daily round of care and toil not only draws more largely than that of the stronger sex on the physical and mental energies, but is lightened by none of that relief which is afforded by a greater variety of duties and more frequent periods of rest.

How the want of suitable amusements can be best supplied; how their prevalent tendency to run into dissipation can be counteracted, are questions not within my province to discuss, but which are worthy of most serious consideration. Whoever will do ever so little towards furnishing a satisfactory answer, will perform an acceptable service to his race.

Another source of mental inefficiency, if not actual derangement, not very uncommon among us, is a want of due relation between our abilities and our aspirations, — between the objects we seek and our means of obtaining them. Some fail of accomplishing their mission by aiming too low, and always gazing on a cheerless, hopeless future. With powers adequate to almost anything, they go through life distrustful of their strength, and recoiling from any determined effort, because, to their feeble faith, it promises no result but discomfiture and disgrace. With every successive year their courage and self-confidence diminish, and with them their disposition to engage in the conflict of life, until finally they abandon the attempt, and passively yield to their fate.

Others, on the contrary, fail by aiming too high. They measure their abilities, less by actual experience of what they can do, than by the allurements that gild their vision of the fu-

ture. Fitted by nature for the humbler walks
of life, they aim for the higher, and the calling
wherein they might have done some service to
their kind is spurned for one that fills a larger
place in the estimation of the world, and requires a larger comprehension than they possess.
If by dint of good fortune they succeed in reaching the coveted position, it is only to find themselves beyond their depth, and to prepare for the
countless mortifications and disappointments
that crown the efforts of aspiring mediocrity.
The effect of such mistaken estimates is prejudicial to the health of the mind, sometimes in
one way, sometimes in another. In some, especially those who are constitutionally susceptible, the repeated failure of their plans produces
a morbid irritability, that, sooner or later, terminates in disease. In others, the mental powers
become paralyzed, as it were, and they slide
through life, in pitiable feebleness and obscurity.*

Another prolific source of mental impairment
among us is our ardent and impulsive temperament. I know not if the fact is to be attributed to atmospherical conditions, to nervous id-
iosyncrasies, or to national manners; but the

* This particular source of mental inefficiency has been admirably described and illustrated by Dr. Edward Jarvis, in *American
Journal of Education*, March, 1858.

fact itself is unquestionable, that, from the cradle to the grave, we are ever in haste. Whatever we do must be done in a hurry. Whether we eat or sleep, work or play, talk, write, or think, it must be accomplished under a pressure of excitement. Nothing in the whole range of our concerns seems to exhibit any exception to this principle. Whether it be a funeral or a wedding, a religious or political enterprise, in every form of business or pleasure, in every manifestation of joy or sorrow, in every plan for accomplishing good to ourselves or our race, the constant thought is how to obtain the maximum result in the shortest possible time. A few months or years seem to be sufficient for any conceivable purpose, and we regard with wonder, if not contempt, the steady perseverance that devotes a lifetime to any object whatever. Of all the qualities which a person or thing can possess, the highest in our estimation is speed. Not how well, but how quick, is our test of merit and measure of regard. The old-fashioned virtues, strength, stability, firmness, are rather respected than admired. The popular plaudits are bestowed upon whatever implies rapidity of conception or of performance; and the national reputation is supposed to be involved, not more in the punctuality with which we meet our pecuniary obligations, or our fidelity in executing the terms of a treaty, than in the feats of our fast horses, fast ships, and fast men. Unquestionably, this trait in our national character tends to precipitate the vital movements of the brain, and consequently to consume its energies faster than they can be supplied. Difficulties and disappointments which are especially incident to hasty and impetuous enterprise, frequently occurring, prematurely rob the mind of its elasticity, and prepare it for early decay. To suppose that the highest possible degree of nervous tension can be maintained for many years without impairing the efficiency of the brain, is simply to ignore the established principles of physiology. What the American brain wants, above all things else, is, as they say of machinery, a steadier movement. The quality of character in which we are peculiarly deficient is that moderation which springs, not from indolence or apathy, but from well-grounded self-confidence and unwavering self-possession.

CHAPTER IV.

MENTAL HYGIENE AS AFFECTED BY THE PRACTICES OF THE TIMES.

HAVING disposed of the particular incidents and events which impair the health of the mind, I now come to those traits peculiar to the intellectual, moral, political, and social condition of our times, which produce a similar effect. Without taking them into the account, it would be impossible to furnish a satisfactory answer to some of the questions which the subject presents.

The present is an age of great mental activity. The amount of it now required for maintaining the ordinary routine of the world would have passed all conception a century ago. Especially is it obvious in that constantly progressive enlargement of the field of industry, whereby the energies of the race have been directed to an increasing variety of pursuits. The kind and degree of mental activity produced in this way, though scarcely perceptible in its minutely divided state, swells at last into an enormous aggregate. When we consider the amount of thought that has been concerned in bringing the manufacture of a pin or a screw to its present state of perfection, we may have a remote conception of the amount of that kind of mental exercise which is required in creating and conducting the countless processes of human industry. Here is no stand-still. Every process intended to subserve the wants or pleasures of man is susceptible of improvement; improvement implies mental effort; and this effort is actually made by a large proportion of those who are engaged in mechanical employments. The class of persons who follow any pursuit with more intelligence than a machine is rapidly increasing, and to this fact we are more deeply indebted for our progress, than to those achievements of master-minds, which, however prolific in results, must be comparatively rare. In those primitive times when successful employment only required a certain acuteness of the senses and faculties common to man and the brutes, disease was not often induced in the brain by an undue exercise of its powers. Neither was mental disease common among those celebrated nations whose literature and art are still synonymous with learning and taste. The throngs that listened with eager ears to the prince of orators, and gazed on the noblest productions of the chisel, felt some stir of emotion, and treasured up for the

15

hours of quiet meditation many an image of beauty and heroic virtue. Peradventure, they may have been led, by the thoughts that breathed and words that burned around them, to some manly resolve or noble endeavor. But they knew little of the mental toil and conflict, the special effort and the steady endurance, which characterize the daily experience of the corresponding classes in our own time, who flock to a political gathering or a popular lecture, with what benefit they may, and gratify their sense of the beautiful in staring at the wax-figures of the museum or menagerie. During the feudal ages, also, the masses had but little occasion to think; it was enough for them to obey. Their intellectual exercise was chiefly confined to the services of religion, and even here they were required to be the passive recipients of the ideas and emotions of others.

These views lead us to the question, whether or not mental diseases are increasing, and it is one of the deepest interest to all who are disposed to believe in the indefinite progress of the race. If, year after year, the amount of human happiness and the capacity of improvement have been seriously diminished by this steadily increasing evil, it is the part of wisdom to learn the fact and provide the remedy. On the question itself, touching the increase of insanity,

opinions have been much divided. Nothing
would seem to be easier than to settle it, by
comparing the number of the insane with that
of the whole population, at periods somewhat
remote from each other. But this supposes a
fact that does not as yet exist. In no part of
the world has a census of the insane been taken,
at two different periods, with any reliable degree of accuracy. Indeed, the attempt has seldom been made at all. Estimates founded on
partial returns, embracing a single district or de-
nomination of people, have been occasionally
made; but, being vitiated by that uncertainty
which must always exist, where inferences take
the place, in some degree, of actual facts, they
can be of little worth in determining any practical question. It deserves notice, however, that
every successive estimate of this kind has
showed a larger proportion of insane than any
previous one. Thus, it has risen, in Great
Britain, from 1 in 7000 to 1 in 300; in France,
from 1 in 1750 to 1 in 1000; in the Rhenish
Provinces of Prussia, from 1 in 1000 to 1 in
600. In the United States, the proportion appears to have risen, during the period between
1840 and 1850, from 1 in 978 to 1 in 738. In
Massachusetts, where the attempt has, several
times, been made with unusual care, to ascertain the number of the insane, the same result

has been observed. In 1847, it was reported to be 1 in 606, and in 1854, 1 in 300. In Rhode Island, the census of 1850 showed the proportion of 1 in 633; while, in the same year, private inquiries found it to be, at the very least, 1 in 351.

These results may only indicate the greater accuracy which repeated investigations generally produce; but if they do not show an appalling increase of the disease, they do show an amount of it, which, a few years since, before its dimensions were so carefully measured, would have been regarded as almost incredible. When we consider, in this connection, the well-authenticated fact, that the prevalence of insanity is proportioned somewhat to the degree of cultivation and refinement which the people have reached, the conclusion seems to be inevitable, that much of it originates in the incidents and conditions peculiar to the civilized state. The laws of physiology might have led us to expect this result. The judicious use of an organ, we know very well, increases its power and confirms its health; but excessive exercise — that which requires an undue share of the vital energies — leads to an unhealthy condition. Every advance in civilization implies additional cerebral effort. The proportion of those who use their brains for anything beyond the ordinary functions of life, is increased by it ; and with this fact is necessarily found another, viz: that the proportion of those who, in one way or another, use their brains immoderately or injudiciously, is also increased. It would hardly seem to require an elaborate investigation to prove that, other things being equal, the mind which only directs the hand in the coarser operations necessary to the mere support of life, will be less liable to disorder than one which feels the spur of higher motives and provides for a higher circle of wants. The brain of the savage partakes of the common exemption from disease shared by his stomach, heart and lungs. It knows little of that severe tension which the civilized man's endures, and which tends to create a morbid ir- ritability easily converted into disease.

We are not to forget, also, that, under the ap- pliances of civilization, the normal hardihood and elasticity of the brain are rather diminished than increased, so that it often fails, less in con- sequence of the magnitude of its efforts, than of its feeble power of endurance. This kind of enfeeblement it shares in common with the other organs, and it would be as idle to deny the fact, as it would to deny that gout, consump- tion, and enlargement of the heart, are indicative of that vital deterioration produced by the luxu- ries and trials of civilized life. It certainly will not be denied that the standard of health has been somewhat lowered among us, during the last fifty years; and such being the case, we have no reason to suppose, other things being equal, that the brain alone has escaped the general fate. But other things are not equal. In addition to the deteriorating influences which affect all the organs alike, the brain, as we have already remarked, is subjected to a strain which has been steadily increasing with the increasing wants and excitements of life. And here we must bear in mind, what is sometimes practically forgotten in discussions of this subject, that the brain is the material instrument, not only of reason, but of the emotions, sentiments, and propensities. Through it come joy and sorrow, the triumph of success, the pang of disappointment, the spur of ambition, the storm of passion, the love of the good and the beautiful, and the peace and trust of religion. Were man merely a reasoning animal, the amount of insanity that might be produced by hard thinking would be comparatively small. And even were we to embrace in this immoderate exercise of his great prerogative, the close and protracted attention often required in his various pursuits, there would still be a large remainder of mental disorder to be traced to some other exercise of mind.

Strangely enough, in the face of this distinction, some persons can see, in the influences of
civilization only the stimulus it affords to the
thinking faculties, and find, as they imagine,
that communities abounding in minds thus exercised will favorably compare, in point of mental health and vigor, with others comparatively
exempt from the labor of thinking. It appears,
for instance, from recent statistics, that the rural districts of England furnish a larger proportion of insane than the manufacturing, and on
the strength of this fact is put forth the doctrine, not altogether new, however, that the increased mental activity which accompanies
every advance in civilization is really favorable
to mental health. " The Hodges of England,"
it is said, " who know nothing of the march of
intellect, who are entirely guiltless of speculations of any kind, contribute far more inmates
to the lunatic asylums than the toil-worn artisans of Manchester and Liverpool, who live in
the great eye of the world, and keep step with
the march of civilization, if they do but bring
up its rear." * This explanation is not quite
satisfactory, because the statement on which it
rests is rather a matter of rhetoric than of actual fact. The toil-worn artisans of Manchester
and Liverpool are, probably, as guiltless of spec-

* *London Quarterly Review*, April, 1857.

ulation as the Hodges of the rural districts. There is nothing in the occupation of making the head of a pin, or driving a steam-engine, more conducive to mental activity than shearing sheep or holding a plough. The extreme division of labor now introduced into most manufacturing processes, and the narrow range of attention consequently allowed to the operative, most effectually preclude any exercise of thought; but the labors of agriculture, with all their supposed monotony, are still not without variety, and, every hour, require the exercise of judgment and discretion. The fact in question has been observed in this country. We have already referred to the fact that in Massachusetts, the rural counties of Berkshire, Hampshire, and Franklin, have a much larger proportion of insane than the manufacturing and maritime counties of Suffolk, Essex, and Plymouth. Nobody here, certainly, would think of explaining this difference by supposing that the mass of the population in the former districts have less intellectual activity than that of the latter. Hodges, no doubt there are, who become insane from mere mental torpidity, but they are not confined to the rural districts. Unquestionably, the number of those who think closely and continuously, seeking to elaborate some new idea, is greater in the commercial and manufac-

turing districts; and this might explain their
comparative exemption from mental disease,
were it the only point of difference between
them. We have only to consider, with some
degree of particularity, the peculiar agencies of
a highly civilized condition, to be quite satisfied
that their tendency is to make large drafts on
the mental energies, and thereby facilitate the
action of more immediate causes of disease.

No single incident of civilization has contributed so much to maintain the mental activity of modern times as the art of printing;
and at no period since its invention have its
benefits and its evils been more widely diffused.
A multitude of mechanical improvements have
so reduced the expense of the process that its
productions are brought within the reach of
every reader in the land, while the proportion of
those who actually read is twentyfold greater,
no doubt, than in any previous generation.
How long is it since, in the interior of the country, a new book was seldom seen among the
smoke-dried volumes that composed the domestic library, and a newspaper was a luxury not to
be rashly indulged in ? People might be stirred
by the prospects of the crops, by an approaching election, or by the appeals of a fiery
preacher, but they scarcely felt the power of a
literature that, in its infinite diffusion, leaves its

mark on every opinion, sentiment, and emotion. The works of standard English writers, which, a few years ago, were confined to the libraries of the few educated men, are now to be found on the shelves of every country shop. Hardly have the products of the British press been laid on the tables of the club-rooms in Pall Mall, when they are on their way to the remotest recesses of the country. Sixty years ago, a pamphlet by Burke on the French Revolution, closely as that great event was connected with our national welfare, found but a handful of readers on this side the Atlantic; while, in our times, on a theme of no immediate interest, a volume of Macaulay, in every shape that the printer's art can devise, is scattered broadcast through the whole length and breadth of the land.

The multiplicity of books and of readers, not only evinces a degree of mental activity which, a century ago, would have been regarded as scarcely within the bounds of possibility, but much of the literature of the day is of a kind not calculated to promote the mental health. It is more or less directly addressed to the lower sentiments of our nature, thereby impairing that supremacy of the higher which is indispensable in a healthy, well-ordered mind. Many people read only to be amused or excited, not to gain useful information, nor to better understand the

great lessons of life. The man whose habitual
reading has strengthened and enlarged his judgment, elevated his aims, enlightened his perceptions of right and duty, and rendered the life to
come a quickening element in his moral experience, is most likely, so far as intellectual culture is concerned, to preserve the normal vigor
of his mind. But he, on the other hand, whose
reading is calculated only to inflame the imagination with pictures of unhallowed enjoyment,
to banish every manly thought and pure emotion, to extend the empire of passion, and induce him to fill his measure of happiness with
things that perish in the using, is weakening all
the conservative principles of his mind, and fa-
cilitating the approach of disease. How much
of the popular literature of the day is designed
to foster a coarse sensuality, comparatively few,
I apprehend, have any conception. Here it is
enough to say that it is accessible to every
reader in the land, and that a large portion of
those whom it attracts will be found among the
young.

A still greater contrast, if possible, is presented by the newspaper press, which, in the
amount of mental activity of one kind or another that it generates, is unsurpassed by all
other literary agencies put together. There is
not a single phasis of human passion, not a sin-

gle combination of its various elements, not a
single development of its slumbering activities,
not a single abnormal deviation from its ordinary channels, not a single manifestation of its
effects on actual life, which is not displayed by
the public press in the strongest colors that an
ambitious rhetoric can give it. And thus, too,
those sad and fearful chapters in human experience, which, though filled with woe to the parties immediately concerned, once were scarcely
known beyond the limits of a little community, are now presented to every reader in the
land, with every circumstance that can add
force or piquancy to the narrative. The columns of a single newspaper, without exaggeration, it may be said, contain more materials for
stirring the sympathies of men, for good or for
evil, than the unwritten lives of countless multitudes. They occupy the leisure moments of
thousands, which would otherwise be given to
listless rest, and furnish inexhaustible materials
for thought or emotion, — the only kind, perhaps, which they ever obtain. The ephemeral
sheet which to-day is, and to-morrow is cast into
the oven, goes forth on the wings of the wind,
scattering its heterogeneous influences upon
every description of person. A murder or a
suicide, a breach of trust or an audacious rob-
bery, committed in the obscurest corner of the

land, is proclaimed to all the world. The details of a disgusting criminal trial, exposing the darkest aspects of our nature, find an audience that no court-room less than a hemisphere could hold; and a tale of railroad or steamboat disaster stirs the blood of the Eastern lumberman in his camp, and of the California gold-hunter in his digging, even before the coroner's jury has rendered the usual verdict, " nobody to blame." The appeals of an aspiring demagogue, the debates of an excited convention, the platform of a political party, exercise the minds of millions, who, without this agency, would have moved on to their dying hour in happy ignorance of them all.

It is a common impression that the newspaper merely ministers to the natural curiosity of men to know what is passing around them; but it has another and a far more important effect. It is not every occurrence, whose communication to the world can be productive of unmingled good. For reasons just given, no small proportion of those which are thrust upon the reader's attention, leave a positively unhealthy impression; and when we consider that, besides the multitudes who, in addition to other reading, never pass a day without looking over a newspaper, there is a scarcely smaller number who read nothing else, we may get some faint idea of the magnitude of this result. The details of vice and crime which occupy so large a space in the daily sheet, repeated day after day, familiarize the mind with their hideous features, and thus blunt the edge of its finer sensibilities. The effect of it all is, that the mind not only becomes careless of moral distinctions, but incapable, in some degree, of perceiving them; its relish for the simply good and beautiful and true is lost, and in its place we find an insatiable craving for what will create a strong sensation, and a positive sympathy, perhaps, with wrong and wrongdoers. By a well-known law of the animal economy, excessive activity of a function leads, at last, to a morbid condition of the organ; and thus it is that this kind of mental activity becomes a prolific source of cerebral disorder, — not of the more palpable forms, such as inflammation or softening, but of a degree of irritability or abnormal erythism which often terminates in overt disease.

The operation of the principle in question is clearly exemplified in the prevalence of suicide, as I have already intimated. In every community are many persons who, from one cause or another, have lost, in some degree, their natural attachment to life. Still, they have no matured nor settled intention of shortening their days. They tolerate life, and they may, perhaps, in consequence of some change of circumstances, and especially of their own mental condition, regain their natural, healthy views of existence. While in this morbid state, however, they are at the mercy of every adverse circumstance, and even of the most trivial impressions. An account of a suicide meets their eye, in the public prints, and absorbs their attention. With a kind of fascination, the mind dwells upon its details, which are related with extreme minuteness, until it has no power to shut them out. Thus the slumbering spark is kindled into a flame, and the resolve is formed to follow the example, either blindly and automatically, or after a course of reflection somewhat like the following: " This man shuffled off the mortal coil when tired of it, and why should not I? The act was easily and speedily performed ; the circumstances are duly chronicled, even to the smallest particular ; for a few days his name is in every mouth; his character, his conduct, his life, are discussed with all the curiosity incident to a nine days' wonder. The same distinction — it is a distinction, though it lasts but a day — I may also achieve. By death, I could obtain what I never have by living." The next day the details of a new suicide are borne to the remotest parts of the land.

The correctness of these views may not be

readily recognized by all, but let it not be supposed, for that reason, that we are fighting with
shadows. The impression made upon the mind
by surrounding influences is, in a great degree,
a matter of temperament and culture; and,
therefore, nothing can be more different than
the impression thus made on different individuals, under circumstances apparently similar.
Within the whole circle of natural phenomena
nothing is more strange, oftentimes, than the
mental experience of one's own neighbor. An
event scarcely noticed by one, is regarded by
another with the deepest concern. An occurrence, which to one suggests only matter of curious speculation, in another touches the inmost
springs of emotion. A popular movement
which is viewed with pity and disgust by one
class of minds, awakens the sympathies of another, and bears them along, willing captives in
its irresistible course. Hence it is, that persons
of a certain culture and moral temper find it
difficult to conceive how the sheet whose contents they scan with more or less indifference,
can be so potent an instrument of agitation to
any description of readers. Nothing in it, unless it may be a change of prices, makes much
impression on them; overlooking, as they do,
the fact, that in those crowded columns which
they dismiss with a glance are details of vice

and crime, upon which many a reader ponders, until the mind is filled with images that cannot be frequently contemplated without danger. The tales of fiction, too, which abound in the newspaper press, often appeal to the coarsest sentiments of our nature, and are prized solely for the thrilling sensations which they excite. Nobody can suppose that such sensations help one to accomplish the true ends of living; and if so, their effect must necessarily be pernicious and unhealthy.

Another trait in the intellectual character of our times has no little influence upon the health of the mind, though its importance in this connection has seldom been duly appreciated. Never before did so large a proportion of the current literature consist of works of imagination, and never before did they, as a class, display so much ability and artistic skill. Much of the literary talent of the time has been turned into this channel. Many a genius who, in a former period, would have expended his powers in producing an epic poem, or a ponderous history, or, peradventure, a formidable folio of divinity, now seeks for honor and immortality in a series of novels. Although, no doubt, some of the richest and ripest talent of the age has been devoted to this class of productions, yet it is evident that, with the increase

16

of demand and supply, there has been a corresponding facility of production. What was once the result of an arduous effort on the part of some veteran like Johnson or Fielding, is now accomplished with the utmost ease and rapidity by the humblest members of the craft of authorship. Young women, hardly arrived at the age of legal majority, put forth books that sell by thousands ; and a host besides, male and female, whom no man can number, contribute to swell the steadily increasing flood that issues from the press.

The above facts indicate another fact, viz. that novels are now read by every description of persons, and by many who read nothing else. The high and the low, the rich and the poor, the learned and the unlearned, the old and the young, men and women, boys and girls, yield alike to the fascination ; some for the sake of amusement and the desire of a new sensation ; some from curiosity to see for themselves what has excited so strongly the interest of others ; and a few for the commendable purpose of becoming acquainted with every form of intellectual manifestation. The records of every popular public library will show, I apprehend, that of the books most called for within a given period, more than half are novels.

The effect of this kind of reading on the men-

tal health is what we have to consider in the
present inquiry. Of course it varies with the
character of each individual mind, and with the
circumstances that accompany it. Generally
speaking, however, there can be no question
that excessive indulgence in novel-reading necessarily enervates the mind and diminishes its
power of endurance. In other departments of
literature, such as biography and history, the
mental powers are more or less exercised by
the ideas which they convey. Facts are stored
up in the memory, hints are obtained for the
farther pursuit of knowledge, judgments are
formed respecting character and actions, original thoughts are elicited, a spirit of investigation
is excited, and, more than all, life is viewed as it
really has been, and must be, lived. A mind
thus furnished and disciplined is provided with
a fund of reserved power to fall back upon when
assailed by the adverse forces which, in some
shape or other, at some time or other, all of us
must expect to encounter. In novel-reading, on
the contrary, the mind passively contemplates
the scenes that are brought before it, and which,
being chiefly addressed to the passions and
emotions, naturally please without the necessity of effort or preparation. Of late years, a
class of books has arisen, the sole object of which
is to stir the feelings, not by ingenious plots,

not by touching the finer chords of the heart and
skilfully unfolding the springs of action, not by
arousing our sympathies for unadulterated, un-
sophisticated goodness, truth, and beauty, for
that would assimilate them to the immortal productions of Shakespeare and Scott; but by
coarse exaggerations of every sentiment, by in-
vesting every scene in glaring colors, and, in
short, by every possible form of unnatural excitement. In all this there is little or no addition to one's stock of knowledge, no elem.. ·+ of
mental strength is evolved, and no one is better
prepared by it for encountering the stern realities of life. The sickly sentimentality which
craves this kind of stimulus is as different
from the sensibility of a well-ordered mind,
as the crimson flush of disease from the ruddy
glow of high health. A mind that seeks its
nutriment chiefly in books of this description is
closed against the genial influences that flow
from real joy and sorrow, and from all the beauty
and heroism of common life. A refined selfishness is apt to prevail over every better feeling;
and, when the evil day comes, the higher sentiments which bind us to our fellow-men by all
the ties of benevolence and justice and veneration furnish no support nor consolation. Let
me not be misunderstood. I do not say that no
one can read a novel without endangering the

health of his mind, for under certain qualifications, nothing could be farther from producing
such a result than this kind of recreation. Who
can number the hours of discomfort and sorrow
which have been relieved of half their burden
by the delightful fictions of Scott? The specific
doctrine I would inculcate is, that the excessive
indulgence in novel-reading which is a characteristic of our times, is chargeable with many of
the mental irregularities that prevail among
us in a degree unknown at any former period.

Much of the mental activity that characterizes
our people arises from the abundant opportunities that are offered for the pursuit of wealth,
and the consequent variety and novelty of the
enterprises undertaken for this purpose. To
follow on in the same path which his father trod
before him, turning neither to the right hand
nor to the left, and perfectly content with a
steady and sure, though it may be, slow progress, circumscribing his wishes and aspirations
within the range of his present pursuits, — this
may be agreeable enough to people of the old
world, but not so to the greater part of those
around us, who are hoping and striving to
make, or greatly advance their fortunes, by
some happy stroke of skill, some nicely balanced
combination of chances, or some daring speculation. The result all can see and admire, but

few know anything of the wear and tear of
mind by which it was achieved, — of the laborious calculations, the anxious moments, the
sleepless nights, the joy of success, the apprehension of failure. Indeed, our ways of doing
business, our notions of property, our ideas of
happiness, all indicate, as strongly as traits of
character can, that a large portion of our fellow-
citizens habitually live and move and have their
being, under an extraordinary pressure of excitement that brooks neither failure nor delay. If
unsuccessful in one attempt, our inexhaustible
resources furnish the means and opportunities
of trying another, while misfortune and disappointment stimulate rather than depress the
mental energies. Competition neither drives a
man from his course, nor abstracts one tittle of
his zeal and activity. With the world before
him where to choose, he asks nothing but a fair
field and no favor, in order to obtain its prizes.
The hygienic effect of this spirit is obvious to
any one accustomed to regard the operations of
the mind from a medical point of view. The
cracking strain of all the faculties most concerned in the management of business, the
hopes and the fears, the joys and the sorrows,
the anticipations of success or defeat, produce
a rapid consumption of the mental energies,
that strongly disposes to disease.

In no country in the world is trade pursued so much in the spirit of mere adventure as in this. Diligence, honesty, and intelligence reap their customary reward, it is true, but they cannot secure it against the numberless mischances that await it, — perils by sea and perils by land; the fraud of one and the misfortune of another. Impulsive dashes at speculation take the place of well-matured, far-reaching plans; and reckless adventure suits the humor of the times better than sober, shrewd calculation. The strongest house looks forward occasionally with fear and trembling to the day when a heavy acceptance becomes due; and the weaker ones expend more ingenuity in devising ways and means for meeting their obligations than in projecting new operations in business. A pressure in the money-market banishes sleep from many a pillow, and the news of every steamer is scanned with gasping eagerness by multitudes. Thus, in countless ways, the mercantile spirit of our times leads to a fitful and feverish activity of mind more destructive to its health than a far greater amount of steady, continuous exertion.

Over and above that mental activity which is excited by the ordinary pursuits of life, there prevails among us a disposition to penetrate into untrodden fields of inquiry; to construct new systems of philosophy and science; to be-

come absorbed in themes of a special and peculiar character; and especially to speculate in
whatever is strange or mysterious, whether in
the natural or spiritual world. People once
thought they might sometimes abide by the
wisdom of their fathers; that some things were
considered as settled, and others as confessedly
beyond the reach of finite intelligence. In this
belief they spared themselves a vast amount of
the mental exercise which characterizes our
times. Of course, there were exceptions to the
rule, but now the case seems to be reversed —
what was once the exception is now almost the
rule. We question everything; we pry into
everything; and we flatter ourselves that we
bring many things to light. Subjects that once
were supposed to be confined to the province of
the learned, and even by them approached with
a modest distrust of their abilities, are now discussed by an order of minds that disdain the
trammels of logic, and care little for the established principles of science. No qualms of
modesty disturb the complacency with which
they discuss the obscurest themes and propound
their theories and systems. With them, all
those laws and agencies of nature which are
confessedly dark and hard to be understood, are
favorite topics of speculation, while the difficulties that encumber them rather inflame their

curiosity than impress them with a becoming
distrust of their powers. Animal magnetism,
biology, communications with the spiritual
world, have raised in multitudes a deeper interest than they ever manifest in those immutable laws of nature, which, if understood and observed, would vastly enlarge the sum of human
happiness. In all our cities and most of our
villages, not a season passes when lectures are
not given on one or all of the above-men-
tioned subjects, to crowds of eager and believing listeners, in many of whom they excite unhealthy meditation, while in not a few, they furnish the single additional element necessary
to produce an attack of disease. I do not
mean by this to say that there are some forms
of truth or of error that ought not to be investigated. If dangerous in any way, so much the
more necessary that their true nature should be
understood and clearly exposed. But subjects
like those just mentioned should be studied
only by a strong and healthy order of minds,
capable of examining their phenomena by the
light of a sound and well-trained judgment, unbiassed by puerile fancies or a blind credulity.
That such has not been the fact, only shows
that those subjects have been more congenial to
a class of persons in whose intellectual life a love
of the marvellous has been a pervading element.

Another trait of our times strongly calculated to produce an unhealthy condition of mind, is the propensity to concentrate the thoughts and interests upon a single idea. Whatever object is deemed worthy of promotion, whether in morals, politics, literature, or religion, that object is thenceforth regarded as of paramount importance, compared with which all others dwindle into insignificance. By the individual it is believed to be the great question of the day, and destined, like Aaron's rod, to swallow up every other. It occupies his thoughts by day, and haunts his dreams by night. In season and out of season, in the newspapers, in the convention, in the legislature, in the social gathering, he pu··nes it with untiring pertinacity, and is always revolving some new scheme for its advancement. He wonders that any one can feel less ardor in regard to his favorite idea than he does himself, and he doubts their benevolence or sagacity; while those, however distinguished for their virtues, who take opposite views, he is apt to charge with dishonorable motives. At last he gets to believe that there is no hope for the race beyond the pale of his little *ism* or *ology*, and in his zeal for propagating it, he is ready to ride rough-shod over the most deliberate convictions and most cherished sentiments of his fellow-men. This habitual confinement

to a very limited sphere of thought tends to in-
vest the favorite idea with a false coloring, if I
may so speak, which distorts its natural proportions and relations, until it finally assumes all
the characters of a delusion. It becomes us all
to beware how we indulge in this besetting
habit of our times. I make no exception in
favor of objects of unquestionable importance,
for the result would not be very different. It is
the complete surrender of the mind to the control of *any* predominant idea, which constitutes
the danger. Truth may have its fanatics as
well as error.

Another characteristic of the time deserving
of notice in this connection, is a remarkable
proneness to excess and exaggeration in its intellectual manifestations. Truth is supposed to
require a high coloring to make it sufficiently
impressive ; while the calm, the plain, the moderate, whether in the subject-matter, or the form
of expression, is apt to be regarded as stale, flat,
and unprofitable. No matter how sound the
principle, or important the application, or correct
the style ; these qualities are well enough in
their place, but to be made really effective, established landmarks must be jostled, shadowy
distinctions set up, and the whole moral sense
agitated with new and unusual emotions. The
object is less to convince than to move ; less to

gratify an earnest spirit of inquiry, than to
startle and excite; while the worth of any intellectual effort is measured solely by the sensation
it produces. Eccentricity is confounded with
originality, and the force of a clear apprehension and an honest sagacity makes less impression than the sparkle and glitter of exaggerated
statement and strange and startling conclusions.
High-sounding words are mistaken for depth of
meaning, extravagance for intensity, and the
feverish heat of a jaded fancy for the fervors of
a true inspiration. Large is the class of people who care less for instruction than excitement; and, looking upon humility as one of
the obsolete virtues, they think more of letting
their own light shine before men than of receiving illumination from others. Instead of learning their duty in the old-fashioned way, from
the counsels of the wise and the precepts of
Scripture, and earnestly striving to perform it,
they start at once as apostles of reform, and woe
to those who question their fitness for the mission. Have we not seen young ladies just
emerged from the restraints of school, scoffing
at the opinions of the world, proclaiming their
independence of authority and prescription,
flouting at everything but their own conceit,
and, without religion, without humility, going
about in search of a God? When the storm of

adversity and trial comes, they drift about at the mercy of the waves, with no anchor beneath, no glimpse of clear, serene sky above them.

In every department of intellectual effort, we witness this peculiar trait of our times. To be popular, philosophy must abound in startling theories, and challenge our strongest and dearest convictions; education must aim at apparently great results, rather than the vigorous growth and symmetrical development of the mental faculties; poetry and romance must lay bare the morbid anatomy of the heart, in order to find the real sources of moral life and the true principles of social organization. Books papers, popular lectures, and too often, I fear the pulpit, all testify of this insatiable craving for excitement, and of the general endeavor to minister to its demands. In the same spirit all progress is thought to be slow that does not advance at a railway-pace, and all ideas to be effete and barren that are not moulded after the fashion of the day or the hour. It cannot be questioned that this fondness of the intense, whether real or mock, is unfavorable to mental health, and has contributed, in some degree, to the increase of insanity among us.

Perhaps nothing is better calculated to foster the kind of mental activity in question, than the

practical working of our republican institutions.
A popular government necessarily implies, on
the part of the people, a degree of attention to
political matters, unknown to those who exercise a more limited power. Almost every man
has a voice in the affairs of the town, in the affairs of the county, in the affairs of the state, in
the affairs of the nation, and they require much
of his time and attention. One day, perhaps,
his mind is strongly exercised with the question
to be decided at the next town-meeting, whether
the town will instruct its representative to vote
for the new liquor-law; the next, he is earnestly
discussing with his neighbors the wisdom of
the county commissioners in laying out a certain road; the next, he is striving hard for his
favorite candidates in the approaching State-
election; and at all times, the presidential election, the doings of Congress, the movements of
parties, are inexhaustible themes of earnest reflection and exciting discourse. How different
from us, in this respect, is every nation in
Europe, even that which approaches us most
nearly, both in blood and political institutions!
There, the public attention may be called once
a year to the election of a mayor, but it is an
even chance whether the individual is allowed
to affect the result directly. At longer periods,
the election of a member of Parliament leads to

animated discussions of the great issues involved in the contest, and the measures of government are viewed with intelligent interest;
but in all this feeling, there is often lacking that
earnestness which springs from the fact, that
he — the individual — is to contribute an active
part to that result, and can help to do or
undo whatever his sense of right or propriety
may dictate. However this may be, the political agitation which is never at rest around
the citizen of a republic is constantly placing
before him great questions of public policy,
which may be decided with little knowledge of
the subject, but none the less zeal — perhaps
with more. In these as well as minor questions, he feels it his duty to be always on the
watch, remembering that " eternal vigilance is
the price of liberty." It is not for him to suppose, in any national crisis or emergency, that
the government will take care of the country,
while he takes care of himself; for he himself is
the government, and he must lift up his voice,
if not in the deliberations of the cabinet, yet in
those scarcely less effective, of the caucus or
the convention. In short, whatever may be the
occasion, he feels called upon to have an opinion of his own ; and free to proclaim it, if he
please, to all the world.

But the mental activity which is excited di-

rectly by free institutions is not confined to political matters. It pervades every sphere of action, every exercise of thought. The almost
complete freedom from restraint, and the independence of foreign control, even in matters of
opinion merely, lead to a certain hurry and im-
petuosity of the vital movements, and to an impatience that seeks for results by extraordinary
effort or superficial methods. Between the
calm, steady, and persevering endeavor, the ad-
herence to routine and prescription, which mark
the European, and the novel, dashing career of
the American, defying all rule and contrary to
all precedent, what a remarkable contrast!
And as if our own particular pursuits and the
practical exigencies of life were not sufficient to
absorb our thoughts and interests, we rush into
every strife and take sides in every question
that agitates the public mind. Nothing is so
remote from our special duties and customary
thoughts, and so clearly within the province of
a professional training, as to deter us from having an opinion of our own respecting it, and
even of making it the basis of practical action.
We have no idea of any division of labor here,
and think ourselves as competent to sit in judgment on questions that have accidentally been
brought before the public notice, as they
who have made them the study of a lifetime.

If, in this way, every man is not precisely his
own doctor, or lawyer, or minister, yet he enters
with the zeal of a partisan into every contest
between rival systems of medicine, law, or divinity. He catches the battle-cries raised by
contending sects, and plunges into the strife
with as much ardor and recklessness as if his
means of living depended upon the result.
How different, in this respect, is the present generation from all the past, in which people were
quite satisfied, sometimes, with taking their
opinions on trust, in the belief that others
might be better qualified by education and experience to form them, than they were themselves, and thereby avoided one fertile source of
that excitement and agitation which prepare
the mind for disease.

Another serious evil of our times, especially
important as being the prolific parent of many
others, consists in the popular views on the subject of education. It will scarcely be denied
that the proper training and development of the
moral powers are necessary to the promotion of
the moral and physical well-being of the individual. The paramount object of education —
that alone which should be recognized as such
in a Christian community — should be to make
good men ; not merely learned men, filled with
various knowledge, but men ever true to the

right, the honorable, the honest, and ever ready
to acknowledge the claims of their fellow-men
upon their sympathy and support.   Indeed, the
necessity of stating such a proposition with any
degree of formality shows, better than anything
else could, the extent of the neglect in question.
The idea almost universally associated with education is that of furnishing the mind with
a certain amount of attainment in various
branches of knowledge ; so much arithmetic,
so much geometry, so much grammar, so much
geography, &c.   If any higher idea than this is
connected with the subject, it is only that of
disciplining the intellectual powers in such a
manner as to fit them better for fresh acquisitions and for the practical business of life.
That every individual has received from nature
certain faculties whose activity and direction
will have an important bearing on his happiness as connected with his relations to his fellow-men, no one doubts ; but the apprehension
that they may not receive their rightful share of
attention in the common modes of education,
seems not to be entertained at all.   To few
comparatively has it ever occurred, that the
training of these faculties is a legitimate object
of education in the popular sense of the term.
To make any proficiency in this or that branch
of knowledge, a course of special instruction by

means of books, teachers, and apparatus, is regarded as indispensable. On the other hand, to
make men pure, benevolent, conscientious, com-
passionate, obedient to God, and faithful to
man, desirable and important as these traits are
universally considered, no special aids of education are recognized and provided.

There remains but one other source which, at
present, could possibly furnish the moral culture
so desirable, — I mean the family, the home.
Here, then, if anywhere, we are to look for that
moral training which is to fit our youth for the
active pursuits of life, and prepare them to meet
its seductions and its duties. Here, if anywhere, they are to acquire the power of govern-
ing passion and resisting the impulses of the
lower appetites ; of discerning the nicer shades
of right and wrong; of sacrificing self to the call
of benevolence or duty; and, amid trial and
change, steadily keeping in view the great ends
and purposes of life. The time has never been
when this kind of training in its highest condition, was very general in our country ; but I
submit, as a matter of fact, whether, imperfect
as it has been, it has not greatly declined during
the last few generations? Unquestionably, at
one time, the domestic rule was needlessly rigid
and disagreeable, and led to an asceticism of
manners equally prejudicial to the mental health

and the moral welfare. At present, however, we have little to fear from this source, the danger all lying in the opposite direction. The asceticism of our ancestors was infinitely less injurious than the license which characterizes the domestic training of their descendants. How many of this generation complete their childhood, scarcely feeling the dominion of any will but their own, and obeying no higher law than the caprice of the moment. Instead of the firm but gentle sway that quietly represses or moderates every outbreak of temper, — that checks the impatience of desire, that requires and encourages self-denial, and turns the performance of duty into pleasure,—they experience only that feeble and fitful rule that yields to the slightest opposition, and rather stimulates than represses the selfish manifestations of our nature. After such a beginning, it could hardly be expected that during the transition period between childhood and manhood, the voice of parental authority would be more faithfully heeded. In the rapidly widening circle of desire, lessons of moderation and temperance make less and less impression on the heart. Amid the selfishness around him, which begins by disgusting and ends in subduing his unsophisti. ⁓ᵈ nature, the youth is little enabled to add new power to the calls of conscience. Enlarged means of

self-gratification strengthen no effort of self-
denial; and in the presence of companions a few
steps farther advanced in the career of indulgence, every manly sentiment is stifled, every
noble aspiration is repressed, until at last, and
long before the age of legal majority, the moral
nature presents a dead level of heartless worldli-
ness. The instructions of school or college may
continue, but less than ever are they applied to
the issues of the heart. The family circle is yet
unbroken, but its moral influence is gradually
enfeebled, because wanting the sanction of authority. The passions become more imperious
with every indulgence, each successive temptation is more faintly resisted, and life begins to
be contemplated, not as a field of discipline and
improvement, but a scene of inexhaustible opportunities for fulfilling hope and gratifying
desire. Could we look into the inmost chambers of the youthful mind, how seldom should
we fail to see an imagination teeming with
unhallowed desires and ambitious schemes, an
impatience of salutary restraint, a self-reliance
that has in it no element of faith, and views of
duty ennobled by no higher principle than that
of selfishness.

The legitimate result of these defects in education is, that finally, the ordinary virtues of life
are degraded to a very subordinate rank. Pa-

tient and persevering industry with its slow and moderate rewards, honest frugality and a temperance that restrains every excess, frequent and faithful self-examination, clear and well-digested views of duty, become distasteful to the mind, which can breathe only an atmosphere of excitement, craving stimulus that rapidly consumes its energies and destroys that elasticity which enables it to arise from every pressure with new vigor and increased power of endurance. It reels under the first stroke of disappointment, and with the loss of those objects on which it had placed its affections, it turns upon itself to revolve some hateful idea, until it becomes a fixed and vivid delusion. And thus it is that many a man becomes insane by exposing himself to extraordinary trial and temptation, with none of those conservative principles which a really good education can impart.

Neither are some of the prevalent views respecting the intellectual education of our youth any better calculated to promote the health of the mind. In the worthiest sense of the term, it means something more than the acquirement of so much knowledge. It falls far short of its highest purposes, when it fails of securing discipline, growth, and strength, among its results. In our anxiety to obtain speedy and tangible results, we manage the education of our children somewhat as we often manage our capital, going upon the plan of quick returns and small profits. They are made to go over much ground in a given time; their accumulations are large and showy, if not solid; but the process whereby this result is accomplished, instead of adding much to the available power of the mind, has often the contrary effect. A strong and well-balanced mind — I leave out of the question great minds, for they are made by nature — a mind capable of clearly discerning the essential conditions of a question, stripped of all accidental and adventitious circumstances; of never confounding the suggestions of fancy or fashion with the deductions of pure reason, cannot be a frequent result of the training so common among us. It may make brilliant and showy men, not incapable, in fact, of producing a sensation in the world; but it will not preserve them from the seductions of fashionable systems in philosophy or morals, nor fit them, in the best possible manner, for the practical exigencies of life. The fact accounts sufficiently for the prevailing disposition to run after novelties, and dwell with absorbing interest on whatever excites a giddy curiosity or stimulates the sense of the marvellous. Under a more rational training, we have a right to suppose that a mul-

titude of objects which now seriously engage
the attention of men, with no better result
than to weaken, if not destroy, every conservative principle in their minds, would never be
entertained, and thus a prolific source of mental
deterioration would be avoided.

The prevalent views on the subject of intellectual training are responsible for much of
the prevalent mental infirmity and inefficiency.
And certainly the cause is perfectly adequate to
the effect. We all recognize the correctness of
the principle in question, in regard to physical
training. We never imagine that the wrestler,
or rower, or runner, can obtain the vigor and
hardihood necessary for success, by sleeping on
down, indulging in luxurious food, and living at
ease. We know that they can be obtained only
by a long-continued, arduous, uncompromising system of training. The growth and development of the mind is subjected to the operation of the same law, but we have had frequent
occasions already to show how little the fact
is recognized. It is worth our while to consider
another error in youthful training, because it is
very common and supposed to be very innocent,
though calculated, beyond any other error, to
impair the future efficiency of the mind. It is
supposed that children are incapable of comprehending books made for the use of grown-up

people, and the idea, fully carried out, at the
present day, of furnishing the youthful understanding with special helps and appliances, in
the shape of juvenile books, is regarded as one
of the great improvements of the age. It is
consummate folly, no doubt, to put into the
hands of a child a book quite beyond his power
of comprehending, but in our endeavor to make
everything simple and easy, to strew the path
of knowledge with flowers, to remove, in short,
every occasion for effort and struggle, we have
erred as far to the opposite extreme.

The world has, probably, never been without
juvenile books since books began to be printed;
but, while in former days they were comparatively few, in the form of some simple tale or
traditionary legend, they are now as " thick as
leaves in Vallombrosa," embracing every topic
supposed to afford materials for instruction or
amusement, and constituting a distinct department of literature. The object seems to be,
either to bring the subject treated nearer the
juvenile comprehension, by simplifying the
thoughts and the language, or to render it
more attractive, by blending with it a little romance, upon Lord Bacon's principle, I suppose,
that " the mixture of a lie doth ever add pleasure." Much of the most respectable talent of
the time is engaged in supplying the demand

for these books, and this supply, joined with that which evinces no talent at all, is devoured by the child, with a rapidity unknown to the tardier movements of riper intellects. Whatever the subject which the progress of knowledge has brought forward, sooner or later it gets into the shape of a book for children, with all the accessory attractions which the ingenuity of the printer, the binder, and the engraver can furnish. Is it desired to acquaint the young pupil with the history of a certain period, or the life of a great man; it would indicate a long distance behind the times, to refer him to those immortal writings in which the events and the actors are described. There is always at hand some little book containing the desired information in miniature, divested of all hard words and troublesome reflections, and, peradventure, invested in the garb of an attractive tale. Is it desired to inculcate some important truth in religion, suitable to guide the life and keep the heart from evil; it is thought that the purpose cannot better be accomplished than by means of a story abounding in incident and adventure, and ending, probably, with love and a marriage. Is a lesson in morals to be stamped on the tender mind; still the never-failing little book will render unnecessary any recurrence to such obsolete authors as Johnson or Paley. Is botany or chemistry, or physics, to be taught; still the means are the same. Even the beautiful simplicity of the sacred oracles has not saved them from being converted into namby-pamby, to accommodate them to the taste of the rising generation, and high dignitaries of the church are not wanting to give their sanction to the deplorable preparation. In short, nothing seems to be too profound, nothing too simple, nothing too high, nothing too ignoble, to be brought within the compass of this class of books. They have come upon the land, like the locusts of Egypt. They are piled up, ceiling-high, on the shelves of every bookstore; they fill the closets and tables of every domestic dwelling, from the hovel to the palace; and, as if they were the most approved means of leading the steps of the young into the paths of virtue, and enlightening their minds with a knowledge of the truth, they form the great staple of every Sunday-school library in the country.

It is a sufficient objection to this juvenile literature, that it vitiates the taste, weakens the understanding, and indisposes and unfits it for a more elevated kind of reading. By having the results of science and art, the lessons of morality and religion, ever presented in the garb of a story, with lively incidents and an agreeable

ending, — vice punished and virtue rewarded,
according to the most approved methods of romance, — the youth imbibes false ideas of the
stern realities of life, and finds the common and
unadulterated truth too insipid to awaken any
interest in his mind. Indeed, these books are
read, or, more correctly speaking, devoured, not
so much for the sake of instruction as amusement; not so much for the principles they may
profess to inculcate, as the incidents and ad-
ventures in which they abound. This result is
just what might have been expected; and I submit to those who have better means of judging,
whether, as a consequence of this result, the
youth of our time do not manifest a marked
unwillingness to give their attention to anything
calculated to excite any activity of the higher
mental faculties. Many a man, I imagine, who
finds his children arrived at their twelfth or thir-
teenth year with no other intellectual furnishing
than such books supply, bethinks himself, all at
once, that long before that age he loved to resort to his father's library, and hang with delight
over the pages of some unwieldy history or
book of voyages; or, in the absence of more attractive material, plunge into the mazes of controversial divinity. The lads of this generation
would stand aghast at sight of the huge folios
and formidable octavos over which their fathers

spent many a Saturday afternoon, laying up
treasures of knowledge as enduring as life.
Their mental aliment must be subjected to a
process of preparation, whereby it is deprived of
its bones and sinews, and seasoned with stimulants to provoke a fastidious and jaded appetite.
If this is a fair statement of the effects that
have arisen from the abundance of juvenile
books, it scarcely admits of a question, whether
the youth of former times were not more
fortunate, who, after having mastered the contents of every book in the house and neighborhood, looked forward with a pleasurable impatience, as Daniel Webster says he and his
brother were accustomed to, to the advent of
the new-year's almanac. I doubt not those
great men derived more benefit from that humble annual than they would from an unlimited
supply of juvenile books; for in less than twenty-
four hours, every line of poetry was committed
to memory, every date fixed in the mind, every
apothegm duly pondered, and every arithmetical
puzzle solved.*

We greatly underrate the youthful intellect in

---

* It will be observed, I trust, that the objection is urged against
the excessive use of juvenile books, without implicating the character of any particular writer. Many an admirable book has been
written for children, and the names of Barbauld, Edgeworth, and
Sedgwick, are associated with memories as profitable as they are
pleasant.

supposing that a special class of books is needful for furnishing it with intelligible and attractive reading. The mistake is the more curious, inasmuch as it occurs by the side of another of the opposite character. The very boys and girls who are practically supposed to be unable to read a history except in a diluted state, are kept, for years together, upon the study of grammar — a science which, even in its elementary state, is of a most abstruse and metaphysical character. And many other school studies, such as geometry, algebra, rhetoric, mental philosophy, require a far greater reach of intellect than many of those works which are the glory of English literature. I believe that those works will furnish an abundance of suitable reading for a youth ten years old and upwards; and no one can suppose that they are not better adapted to improve the taste and cultivate the higher powers of the mind than the juvenile books of the day. He may not perceive, at every step, the keen sagacity of Gibbon, nor fully appreciate the quiet graces of Prescott and Irving, but he will learn on good authority the facts of history, and feel somewhat of its grandeur and dignity. He may not perceive the full significance of Shakespeare's greatest thoughts, nor be charmed with the harmony of Spenser's verse, " in lines of linked

sweetness long drawn out," but he will catch
an occasional glimpse of the clear upper sphere
in which the poet moves, and fix in his mind
many an image of purity and loveliness, of
tried virtue and high-souled sacrifice, that will
preserve it, in some measure, from the contami-
nation of ignoble thoughts and desires. I think
no one will maintain that boys or girls twelve
years old, of fair parts and tolerably educated,
are incapable of understanding and enjoying
the greater part of Addison, Pope, Goldsmith,
Robertson, Hume, Cowper, Burns, Southey,
Macaulay, Scott, and Crabbe. And yet how
many such youth there are, who never read beyond a page or two of these authors, nor even
heard their names! Indeed, if a person, recol-
lecting the delightful hours they furnished him
when first gratifying his love of intellectual
pleasures, should propose them to the youth of
this generation, he would be likely to be regarded with a look of curiosity, as a man born
out of due time, or, at any rate, quite behind
the age which has provided more suitable aliment for the tender mind, in the preparations of
Peter Parley and his prolific school. This is
a serious matter and well-deserving attention;
but I can only say, in conclusion, that we may
carry our systems of school-instruction to the
highest point of perfection, yet, so long as the

juvenile literature of our times maintains its present place in the popular estimation, it will be in vain to expect a generation of vigorous, self-relying, healthy minds. Important, however, as all this is, it is but incidental and subordinate to a point of still greater importance.

The habit of reading books that excite but little activity of thought becomes too strongly fixed to be weakened by the higher aims and purer tastes of riper years. The youth has read, not that he might learn to think, but that he might be amused, and as the appetite only grows by what it feeds upon, increase of years produces no change in the object of his reading. True, the books of children have lost their wonted power to charm ; but now their place is supplied by another and far more objectionable kind. The faculty of the mind chiefly addressed in both is the imagination, or that power which forms ideal creations abundantly endowed with those incidents and attributes that constitute the greatest charms in actual realities. In earlier years, the pleasure thus obtained is undoubtedly innocent though enervating, and has in it no taint of sin. But at the later period we are now considering, a change has come over the whole spirit of the youth. A new order of emotions, desires, and aspirations has arisen within him, and a veil has been lifted

from before his vision, disclosing creations of
exquisite loveliness whose earthly types are ever
near to enliven his conceptions and give them
an almost objective existence. The relations of
the sexes, scarcely thought of before, have become the predominant subject of his thoughts,
and he feels the witchery of an irresistible spell
stealing over his senses, and polarizing, if I may
borrow a term from physical science, the very
fountains of his being. To meet this state of
things, to touch the chord that nature has
strung, apparently, for the very purpose, there
has appeared the description of publications
just alluded to. Although their predominant
features are love and romance, they have few
points in common with the works of the great
masters of fictitious writing. Although the
course of true love is a constant ingredient of
the latter, yet it is often subordinate to a
higher object, and the impurities with which it
is associated are indicative of bad manners
rather than bad morals. , But censurable as
the works of some of the older writers undoubtedly are, on this score, they are altogether
too tame, too much hampered by a decent respect for decorum, to fulfil exactly the object in
question, — that of stimulating the passions of a
tender mind enervated by vicious training, and
kindling with new and untried desires. Though

embracing much that deserves no stronger epithet of censure than foolish or frivolous, yet the greater part of this kind of literature is calculated, if not designed, to debase the tone of moral sentiment, to suggest impure ideas, and send forth the imagination to wander into unhallowed paths.

Now let us consider the youth in that transition period which separates boyhood from manhood. His mind has become enfeebled by an incessant repletion of juvenile literature, and is unconscious of any manly thoughts or lofty aspirations gained by communion with a higher order of intellect than his own. In this condition the allurements of sense are spread before him in every variety of form, and his ear is open to every siren song that floats upon the breeze. He has much leisure, which his tastes dispose him to occupy with reading, and when we consider his previous habits and the present epoch of his life, we cannot be surprised that he should make the acquaintance of this description of books, and abandon himself, body and soul, to their allurements. I say advisedly, body and soul, for the mischievous effects are as obvious and as ruinous upon the one as they are on the other. By a law of our constitution, violent mental emotions thrill through the bodily frame, and this participates in the vital movement. Here, body and mind act and react on each other, and often, so far as the final result is concerned, it seems to be immaterial whether the first impression be made on one or the other. In these books, the tender passion is presented with none of those refinements with which it is associated in pure and cultivated minds. It is designedly made carnal and provocative of impure desire, and the youth who surrenders himself to its seductions becomes thenceforth a stranger to every manly sentiment, while his imagination revels in a world of sense, filled with the charms of a Mahommedan paradise. From this point there is but one step, it is true, to actual, overt licentiousness; but a lingering feeling of shame, a faint sense of responsibility, and a timidity natural under the circumstances, often hold him back from taking that step, and he is contented to indulge in secret, with such means as nature has provided. Month after month, year after year, are spent in this dreamy existence, the unholy flame constantly nourished by the kind of reading in question, and its debasing effects as constantly assisted by the habit of self-indulgence. Sooner or later there begins a series of pathological phenomena which, with more or less rapidity, but usually covering a period of years, conduct their miserable subject to mental and physical ruin. I forbear to dwell on the details of this fearful condition, — the muscular system falter-ing under the least exertion, and constantly op-pressed by a sense of lassitude and fatigue; the nervous system overcharged with irritability, af-fected by the slightest emotion, and turned into a source of weariness and pain; the mind tor-tured almost to distraction by groundless anx-iety and self-reproach, harassed by a sense of guilt, and vague apprehension of a future dis-closing not a single ray of hope, and revolving thoughts of suicide, as the only means of escap-ing from the ever-gnawing worm. Neither would I dwell upon the more common phasis of this condition: the cloud of delusion that rapidly envelopes the whole mind and distorts all its relations; the utter loss of the power of connected thought; the suspicions, jealousies, and ungovernable impulses that precipitate the individual into some fearful act of violence; and that final brutalization of our nature, where, for years together, no spark of humanity gleams through the loathsome prison-house of flesh. But I implore the teacher and the parent to think of these things, and prevent, as they prob-ably may, an evil which they cannot cure. Could they witness occasionally, as I do every day, the melancholy results that may be fairly attributed to that kind of mental training which

stimulates the imagination and the lower moral
sentiments, they would not suspect me of repre-
senting an infrequent accident in the light of a
great and wide-spreading evil. In every hospital
for the insane there may be seen a form of disease preëminently loathsome and difficult of
cure, many cases of which, I doubt not, may be
traced to the kind of reading in question. How
many a noble intellect that once gave promise
of the soundest fruit has thus been blasted, and
with it the hopes, the pride, the solace, of many
loving hearts, the world generally has but little
conception.

From what has been said, it cannot be
doubted that the people of our times live in
an atmosphere of excitement, which, without
the most prudent management, is calculated to
impair the vigor of the mind and facilitate the
invasion of disease. In order the better to estimate the psychological effects of this general
fact, it may be well to contemplate some of the
phases of that remarkable change which has
come over the whole face of society, within the
last fifty or seventy-five years. Take, for instance, as particularly applicable to our purpose, the family of a mechanic, or farmer, or
small trader, in some country town of New
England, at the beginning of that period, and
compare it, in regard to its mental movements,

with such a family at the present time. The ex-
penses of a growing household, and the natural
desire of making some provision for the future,
require, on the part of the elders, unremitting
toil. Their labors commence with early dawn,
and are prolonged into the shades of evening.
They have neither leisure nor inclination to be-
stow many thoughts upon anything far beyond
the circle of their customary pursuits; and their
happiness consists chiefly in witnessing the accumulation of their worldly stores and cultivat-
ing the domestic affections. Outward sources of
gratification are too few to furnish much relief
to the monotony of their daily life. Social intercourse is limited by the same necessities that
confine them to their homes and their labors.
Besides the Sabbath and the national holidays,
they recognize no interval of rest or relaxation;
and an excursion or picnic, or any other con-
trivance solely for the purpose of pleasure, is an
event seldom recorded in their calendar. They
go to meeting on Sunday, where tired nature
often claims her rights, while the preacher plods
along from firstly to seventeenthly through the
beaten track of old New England divinity.
When work is not too pressing, the legal voters
in the family attend the elections, and with the
performance of this duty all farther thought
respecting the politics of the day is dismissed.

Their patriotism needs not the aid of mass
meetings or torch-light processions. No fears
of a crisis, nor the agitations of a civil conflict,
disturb their peace, and however an election
may go, they never doubt that the world will
move on very much as before. The mother is
fully occupied with family cares, but her simple
wants and moderate wishes urge her to no toils
beyond her strength. Labor is the law of her
being, beneficent and salutary, like all other
natural laws, rather than a dire necessity that
must be met at whatever cost. The sons and
daughters share in the domestic duties, except
during the two or three months in winter, when
they attend school to obtain the little learning
that satisfies their wishes. They have but little
more social intercourse than their elders; and a
militia-muster, a husking, or a sleigh-ride, once
a year, constitute their sole means of relaxation.
Their willing feet may, occasionally, have made
the acquaintance of the dance; but the idea of
a theatre or an opera or a concert exists for
them, only in the pictures of the imagination.
They never puzzle themselves about their mission in life, but quietly perform their daily duty,
and lie down at night to enjoy long and sound
repose. Unaccustomed to the refinements of
civilization, and braving every day the rigor of
the elements, they retain unimpaired, for the

most part, the natural vigor of their constitution ; and when the shock of adversity comes, they stand it without going mad or committing suicide. A newspaper is seldom seen in the house, and the advent of a letter makes an epoch in the family history. The domestic library is limited, probably, to Bunyan's Pilgrim, Pike's Arithmetic, Watts's Hymns, a tract or two on controversial divinity, and a half-dozen more, perhaps, of well-thumbed volumes which by some lucky chance have drifted within their precincts. No great questions of the day exercise their wits, and no fashionable follies have turned their heads or impaired their health. They are contented with small gains, and if visions of wealth and magnificence sometimes rise before them, they seldom endeavor to turn them into practical reality. They are not exempt from disease; but it is far more likely to be a fever or a rheumatism, than an affection of the spine, a dyspepsia, or insanity.

How different from all this the circumstances of a family occupying a corresponding position in the social scale, at the present day. No possible arrangement can keep it without the vortex of excitement which draws into its circling eddies every living mortal. Its members, each and all, have much to think of besides their accustomed labors, which, with the males, are

supposed to be limited by an ordinance of
Providence, if not by the laws of man, to just
ten hours a day, or less.   The domestic circle is
entirely too small to bound their affections,
their interests, or their wishes.   The head of the
family has felt the desire of distinction, and
sought the favor of his fellow-townsmen.   He
aspires to a seat in the legislature, or a place on
the board of selectmen, and his political advancement has become to him a source of much
anxiety and care.   He attends conventions for
nominating candidates, and the results of the
elections are watched with the deepest interest.
In the affairs of the religious society with which
he is connected, he may be an active mover;
and on the various points that require to be settled from time to time,—such as the painting of
the church, the purchase of an organ, or the dis-
mission of the minister,—he is sorely exercised by
the diverse views of his fellow-worshippers.   He
is always ready to discuss great questions, and
whether it be a matter of politics or religion, he
has an opinion of his own, and is glad of an opportunity to defend it.   The partner of his
bosom looks well to the ways of her household,
but she has an eye to other ways than these.
The narrowest means and the severest toil do
not entirely repress the risings of an ambition
excited by the display of superior luxury and

leisure around her. She finds that the public has claims on her attention which she is perfectly willing to meet. As often as once a week, at least, there is a meeting of some charitable society, which she is bound to attend, and at no less frequent intervals, subscriptions are to be collected for some favorite object, or a poor family to be looked after, or a special effort to be made for some extraordinary purpose. Her worldly views, too, are more aspiring than she is, probably, willing to admit, and the settlement of her children is a fruitful source both of pleasing and painful emotions. The sons quit the shelter of the parental wing at an early period, and rush to the principal marts of business, where a happier fortune seems to await them. The quiet monotony of their country home is exchanged for the bustle and hurry and change always incident to the struggle for success in the great thoroughfares of life. To be contented with the gains of common, plodding industry, would betray an ignoble spirit, not in accordance with the times, and so they enter upon a restless, uneven career. No doubt, their wits are sharpened by the collisions that attend it, but the draft which is made upon their nervous energies by this incessant strain of the faculties would suffice, a half-dozen times, for all the exigencies of the life of a hum-

ble farmer or mechanic, a half-century ago. It
may not end in positive insanity; but it produces in their offspring, if not in themselves, a
degree of nervous irritability that may easily be
converted into overt disease. The daughters,
too, contract very different habits and entertain
very different views of life from those which
prevailed in their grandmothers' time. Domestic duties may not be despised, perhaps; but
they are endured rather than enjoyed, and, unwelcome as they are, they are relieved by many
a solace not dreamed of in former times. The
family library is no longer the meagre and
musty collection just described, but it contains
some of the classics of the language, albeit the
yellow-covered literature of the day constitutes
its predominant ingredient, and distils its se-
ductive poison into their eager imaginations.
The facilities of travel bring within their means
the agreeable pastime of visiting distant friends,
and even tasting the delights which the crowded
city alone can furnish to gratify the senses and
imagination. A new world discloses its glories
to their admiring gaze, and who shall estimate
the amount of emotion, of one kind or another,
which it kindles! Vague, indefinite longings
for something beyond their reach, a restless impatience of the humble realities of their lot, an
impotent straining for the glittering prizes of

life — these have become a part of their daily moral experience, and exert their legitimate effect on the health of the mind. Let us carefully consider these two phases of our domestic and social life, observing the very different manner in which the nervous system is tasked under each of them, and we shall then understand how it is that, with every advance in civilization, we increase our proneness to nervous disease.

CHAPTER V.

MENTAL HYGIENE AS AFFECTED BY TENDENCIES TO DISEASE.

To those who have unfortunately inherited a predisposition to mental disease, and especially those who have already suffered an attack, the course and conduct of life most likely to prevent its development must be a matter of the deepest concern. While one thus constituted should, certainly, avoid undue anxiety on the subject, yet it would be an error no less serious to ignore the fact altogether, and act precisely as if it did not exist. It would be the wiser thing, to believe that it depends very much on himself, whether or not the morbid germ is to be developed into fatal activity, or kept for many years, if not for life, in a latent condition. Though I would not deny that sometimes the disease is developed, apparently, by no exoteric agencies whatever, yet it is a matter of common observation, that this result is often attributable to incidents and conditions that might have been avoided. There is also reason to believe that many persons, thus unhappily constituted, have warded off an attack of disease, by looking the evil firmly in the face, and resolutely shunning, in their diet, regimen, habits, occupations, amusements, mental and bodily exercise of every description, whatever might be supposed likely to produce unhealthy excitement.

The first consideration I would urge on this class of persons is, that a tendency to mental disease is liable to be increased by any derangement of the bodily health. Wherever its principal seat may be, the brain is liable to be finally involved in the morbid process. I do not mean that a fever or an influenza, a hemorrhage or a broken bone, may be always avoided by any practicable degree of prudence or forecast; and yet it can scarcely be questioned that a very large proportion of our bodily ailments proceed from ignorance, or imprudence, or wilful folly. The proper care of our bodily health, important enough under any circumstances, becomes doubly so when rendered necessary to preserve the health of the mind. Parents who have reason to fear the existence of hereditary mental infirmities in their offspring, have an additional inducement to watch over their health, to strengthen their bodily powers, and promote a happy balance of the various faculties of the mind. It would be unnecessary to dwell on those dietetic rules applicable to all sorts and conditions of youth.

My present object will be best met by directing attention to principles and practices most suitable to such as may be supposed to have inherited tendencies to mental disease.

Although insanity seldom makes its appearance in childhood, yet it can hardly be doubted that the initiatory step is often taken at this period towards the development of morbid tendencies, even when, to the superficial observer, everything indicates high health and a vigorous constitution. In the physical education of this description of children, it should be a prominent object to strengthen the nervous system, — to render it less excitable, and increase its power of endurance. Whatever conflicts with this object, we may be sure is wrong, and nothing calculated to promote it should be neglected. Much sedentary employment, much confinement to warm rooms, sleeping on feathers — all improper enough under any circumstances — are peculiarly adapted to foster susceptibilities to nervous disease. Under their influence, outward impressions are more keenly felt, nervous irritability accumulates, and abnormal movements are more easily induced. Attacks of bodily disease meet with less resistance, and even when apparently thrown off, leave behind them a diminution of the vital forces, and consequently an increased susceptibility to noxious agencies. On the other hand, considerable exercise in the open air, with some disregard of atmospherical conditions, serves to expend the surplus nervous energies, and thus excite a healthier activity in the nervous system. Upon no class of children does the hot-house management operate more unfavorably than on that we are here considering. Upon no other class of children do labor and exposure, properly regulated, prove more salutary; and parents cannot make a greater mistake than to lavish upon them the tenderest nursing.

Of more importance, however, than all this, is the mental and moral training, — or, more strictly speaking, the education and exercise of the brain. This must be managed with paramount reference to its health, to which every other consideration should be subservient. This, of course, requires prudence and discretion, a disregard of the more attractive objects of education, and a superiority over the vulgar prejudices so prevalent on this subject. Whatever habits or exercises are calculated to impair the mental health of any child, must necessarily favor the growth of morbid tendencies wherever they exist. Errors which may be harmless to such as are happily organized, act with fearful effect upon those who have inherited a proclivity to disease. The most pernicious, and, at the same time, the most common of these errors in our present methods of education, is to require an excessive amount of study. It is curious how few have any other idea of the youthful brain, than that of a machine exempted from the ordinary lot of wear and tear. The anatomist has displayed in some degree the wonderful arrangement of its delicate tissues, and traced its progressive development in the ascending orders of the animal kingdom; and the physiologist has shown, by curious experiments, how its vital movements are sensibly quickened by mental emotions; and yet the relation between these facts and the work of education is seldom discerned. On the contrary, the few who do see it and insist upon its practical importance, are often, if not generally, regarded as fanciful and crotchety.

We have already seen that children are made to study while yet too young, and we scarcely need repeat that at the age of three, four, or five, the brain has not acquired the hardihood requisite for study. It may then receive impressions, and the skill of the teacher may turn them to some useful purpose; but any formal exercise of the intellectual faculties is unnatural, and, for the most part, unpleasant. Most young children, fortunately, have too little fondness for study to be injured by it; but there are a

few, of precocious development, to whom it is
never tiresome nor disagreeable.. Encouraged
by fond, mistaken friends, they make wonderful acquisitions ; but in the very bloom of their
promise, they suddenly fail and wither away.
It is at a later period, when the common re-
pugnance to study is overcome by its glittering rewards, that the danger begins. By one
motive or another, the brain is stimulated to an
amount of application that would be excessive
in adult age. The requirements of teachers,
the love of distinction, the thirst for knowledge,
blunt the sense of fatigue, and the usual ignorance or carelessness of nature's laws utters no
warning against the danger. Six, eight, ten
hours a day, in school or out, the mind is engaged in the most exhaustive exercise, and even
the night is not entirely given to rest. If anything is calculated to foster unhealthy tendencies, it certainly is such management as this,
because it vitiates and weakens those energies
on which we must chiefly rely, in maintaining
the health of the brain against the influence of
abnormal conditions.

Supposing the individual who has inherited
tendencies to mental disease, to have arrived at
manhood and entered on the serious business of
life, how shall he prevent, if possible, the development of those tendencies into actual disease ?

Of the danger there can be no doubt; but very
few are aware of it, or care to govern themselves with regard to it. Occasionally, there is
one who sees the prospect clearly before him,
and is sincerely anxious to conform his conduct
to such rules as the nature of his case implicitly
requires. To such, a word of counsel is offered,
in the hope that, if duly heeded and carried into
daily practice, it may avert a calamity that might
justly appal the stoutest heart.

The necessity of ordering one's life with reference to this constitutional defect being admitted, it must be premised that the same
rules of living are not equally applicable to all
men. Difference of temperament, of education,
of taste, of pursuits, require diversity of management ; insomuch that a course of living
most salutary to one might be filled with danger to another. To enjoin upon one who delights in religious gatherings, greater devotion
to spiritual exercises and contemplations, would
be as inappropriate and mischievous, as to caution a man who never enters a church against
undue indulgence in religious emotions. The
reverse of such advice would be most suitable
to each. Every one, therefore, must study his
own case, and ascertain, if possible, where his
peculiar danger lies. There are a few general
rules, however, of universal application.

Most persons have some weak point in their physical constitution, and this, by a well known law of the animal economy, is the first to suffer under any general disturbance of the vital actions. Whatever habit or indulgence, therefore, may be supposed, under the common rules of hygiene, to impair the vital energies, should be carefully shunned. Good habits of living, abundant exercise in the open air, unstinted sleep, plain, nutritious food, moderation and temperance in all things, beneficial as they are to all, are peculiarly important to those whose hereditary tendencies expose them to mental disease. Especially are stimulants, and whatever else is calculated to affect the nervous system, to be used with extreme caution. I do not say that they are invariably and unconditionally injurious, but that they generally are when used to excess, and often are, even when used with judicious moderation. Nobody, therefore, with the morbid tendencies in question, and sincerely desirous of preventing their development, will hesitate to deny himself all indulgence in tobacco and spirituous liquors, not implicitly required by some other conditions. Though not among the most potent agencies in creating insanity where no hereditary predisposition exists, yet few are more efficient than the latter in developing the latent germs

of the disease. This caution is peculiarly necessary, in view of the very common use of these
articles at the present time, — so common as to
be regarded by a large portion of the race as
one of the normal habits of modern life.

Excessive bodily exertion, by deranging some
of the functions of organic life, may thus indirectly occasion mental disease, and therefore
should be cautiously used by the class of persons in question. I have already adverted to
the fact that no small amount of insanity in
this country, especially among the young, married, American women of the humbler classes,
is produced by a degree of daily toil greatly
beyond their power of endurance, and unenliv-
ened by sufficient recreation or amusement.
That the health of our women has been depre-
ciating during the last forty or fifty years, is a
fact too lamentably patent to be questioned.
To be exempt, for a twelvemonth, from some
bodily ailment, or that kind of delicate health
which is but a slight 'remove from it, has
become a fact of no common occurrence.
When persons thus constituted are forced, by
the circumstances of their position, beyond
their strength, it is not strange that, where predisposition to disease exists, the brain should
become the suffering organ. They contribute
very largely to swell the number of cases

charged to " ill-health," in the table of causes
which forms a portion of most of our hospital
reports, — a number which has been steadily
increasing, until it predominates over every
other. The evil is so much the more deplorable, as it seems to be beyond the reach of
any practicable remedy. A single morbific
agency might be met and overcome; but
when the evil results, as it does in this case,
from a host of adverse agencies, — a climate
changeable, and presenting the extremes of
temperature, unventilated apartments, food of
poor materials and badly cooked, patent med-
icines, (become almost as common as daily
bread,) deficient exercise at one time and excessive labor at another, social habits in which
the gratification of the cheerful emotions has
but little place, hereditary tendencies to disease
inexorable in their operation, though utterly
ignored by the mass of mankind, — it needs
a sanguine faith in human docility to expect
any immediate improvement.

However important may be the physical regimen of persons predisposed to mental disease,
it is, unquestionably, upon their mental exercises that the fate of the larger portion must
chiefly depend. How these shall be ordered so
as to best secure the object in view; what kind
and amount of mental application shall be

allowed ; what moral and intellectual powers shall be cultivated or neglected, — these are questions to be carefully and intelligently considered. In fact, no one, with the tendencies in question, has a right to expect immunity from the threatened danger, who has not so considered them, and, as the result of his inquiries, adopted some special rules of living. For this purpose, a few practical hints may be of service, founded upon considerable observation of abnormal obliquities and morbid tendencies.

By the class of persons whose case we are here considering, no more conservative agency can be had than that of suitable and steady employment. Absolute rest, idleness, freedom from care and duty, are not the things most conducive to mental health. Activity is the law of our mental, as well as physical life, and it is not annulled by the presence of morbid tendencies. It requires only to be skilfully modified to be followed by its ordinary results, — continued strength, buoyancy, and endurance. Whatever employment be adopted, it should fulfil certain indispensable conditions.

It should require an amount of application much less than that deemed safe and proper in more happily constituted minds. Here the brain is peculiarly sensitive to any strain upon its energies, and being deprived of its proper

elasticity, it fails to recover itself completely
when the tension is removed. A degree of irritability, and perhaps of discomfort, is finally
established, which may be readily converted
into disease. A full amount of mental labor,
therefore, is out of the question, and it is the
part of wisdom to recognize the fact and conform to its requisitions.

The employment should be not merely an
easy sort of drudgery or busy idleness, but one
as interesting and useful as practicable, and
adapted to the person's taste and station. Simple occupation of the attention is better than
nothing, but it lacks those conservative influences which flow from the consciousness of
having accomplished something that needed to
be done. It should involve no great responsibility, nor subject one to unpleasant intercourse
with others. It should furnish little occasion for
the control of temper, and be as free as possible
from disappointments and failures. There are
many kinds of employment in which these persons might safely engage while the sea is
smooth and the winds light, but which, in
those periods of storm and tempest that are
sure to happen sooner or later, would be full of
peril. If they consult their own welfare, they
will never undertake to command ships, super-
intend railroads, or embark in mercantile speculations.

From social pleasures of the simple, quiet kind, the happiest effect may be expected; but absolute seclusion should not be more carefully avoided than gatherings of people where the sound of passion is heard, and the heart and the will are carried away captive by the irresistible power of sympathy. I do not say that there are no exceptional cases, but, until satisfied by competent authority that the general rule does not apply to them, these persons had better act habitually on the conviction that such scenes are not for them.

Of any employment or recreation, it should be an indispensable condition, that it should not curtail the proper allowance of sleep, either by encroaching on its regular hours, or by filling the mind with thoughts and images that refuse to depart at bidding. Deficient sleep is a source of imminent peril, and when it continues for many days, the appropriate remedies should be sought without delay. A large portion of the secondary attacks of mental disease are occasioned by loss of sleep, induced by circumstances more or less under the control of the patient. No call of duty or of pleasure, whether it be to watch with the sick, or join the festive circle, should be allowed to shorten the period that rightfully belongs to nature's sweet restorer.

When the morbid tendency begins to show

itself, merely in unusual restlessness, there
may be a craving for amusements and exciting scenes, which friends are too ready to
indulge, with no idea of the danger they incur. Nothing can be more mischievous than
such indulgence, calculated, as it is, to cherish
the kindling spark and fan it into an uncontrollable flame. In this condition, quiet, seclusion from gatherings of people and from all
scenes whatever which leave vivid impressions
upon the mind, are implicitly required, distasteful as the discipline may be. These periods of
abnormal excitability may frequently occur in
such persons, and it depends very much on the
firmness and intelligence with which they are
managed, whether they are kept within endur-
able limits, or pass into overt, uncontrollable
disease.

Persons predisposed to mental disease should
carefully avoid a partial, one-sided cultivation
of their mental powers, — a fault to which their
mental constitution renders them peculiarly liable. Let them bear in mind that every prominent trait of character, intellectual or moral,
every favorite form of mental exercise, is liable
to be fostered at the expense of other exercises
and attributes, until it becomes an indication of
actual disease. Here lies their peculiar danger,
that the very thing most agreeable to their taste

and feelings is that which they have most to
fear. Many of this class of persons possess a
large endowment of the ideal faculty. They
delight to dwell in the regions of fancy, and the
subjects they habitually contemplate are such
as the imagination only can supply. From
this prolific source they draw the sustenance of
their intellectual life; and though they may not
necessarily possess a poetical temperament, yet
their duties, their prospects, even the great purposes of life, are apt to be regarded from an
ideal point of view. Severer exercises of mind
— such as require the reasoning powers —
are uncongenial, and consequently neglected.
Close observation, exact knowledge, diligent
application, careful induction, form no part of
a mental experience which is crowded with
strange combinations of thoughts, with beautiful imagery, and all the heterogeneous offspring
of fancy. Thus, the rightful balance of the
intellectual faculties, essential to the highest
health and vigor, is finally lost, and but little
is then required to induce unequivocal disease.
Such persons should beware how they yield to
their favorite contemplations. As a matter of
safety, they should cultivate those faculties
which are concerned with objective or definite
truths, such as those of mathematics, natural
history, and natural philosophy. These require

a more equal and steady attention, and are marked by more exact and tangible results, all well calculated to check that roving movement of the mind, which, under whatever name it may pass, weakens its powers of self-control, and thus invites the approach of disease. Percival, the poet, who, no doubt, described his own experience when he said, —

> " A thousand 'wildering reveries led astray
> My better reason, and my unguarded soul
> Danced, like a feather, on the turbid sea
> Of its own wild and freakish fantasies," —

was, all his life, hovering on the verge of insanity, from which he was saved, probably, by his taste for the study of natural science and of the languages, to which, fortunately, his attention was early directed. They drew his mind from a too intense contemplation of the ideal world, where it was at the sport of every erratic, morbid, vital movement, and fixed it upon truths that required its calm, clear, and steady insight.

The near alliance of the poetical temperament with insanity has passed into a proverb, and, exaggerated though the fact may be, there is much reason to believe that it is not entirely an error. " Perhaps," says the great historian of our time, " no man can be a poet, or even enjoy poetry, without a certain unsoundness of mind."

Without troubling ourselves to discuss the psychological accuracy of this statement, we may fairly maintain its substantial correctness. No one can have witnessed the phenomena of insanity on a large scale, without being struck with the many points of resemblance between the mental movements of the insane and those of the poet whose

> " —— eye, in a fine frenzy rolling,
> Doth glance from heaven to earth, from earth to heaven ;
> And, as imagination bodies forth
> The forms of things unknown, the poet's pen
> Turns them to shapes, and gives to airy nothing
> A local habitation and a name."

In both, the judgment, or the faculty by which ideas or associations are regarded according to the relations of cause and effect, of means and end, ceases to exert its influence, and the thoughts succeed one another, without any very obvious bond of connection besides that of similitude or contrast. In both, the ideal faculty predominates over every other in giving shape and direction to the thoughts, and both are characterized by an intensity of conception unknown to other conditions of mind. This analogy is not stated for the purpose of detracting from the dignity of the poetical character, but that it may give additional force to the warning

against the unlimited and unregulated exercise
of the ideal faculty. Let a man of an unhealthy
mental constitution implicitly yield to its domi-
nation, and allow it habitually to give shape and
direction to his thoughts, and there can be no
hesitation in saying that he is in peril of mental
disease. And it is immaterial, in a hygienic
point of view, whether the trait in question
manifests itself in poetical reading and writing,
in the ideal coloring which invests every object
of contemplation, or in the dreamy reverie which
constitutes the usual mental exercise.

There is another disposition of mind to be
carefully shunned by the class of persons in
question, — that of allowing the attention to be
engrossed by some particular interest to the
neglect of every other, even of those most nearly
connected with the welfare of the individual.
The caution is especially necessary in an age
whose intellectual character is marked by strife
and conflict, rather than calm contemplation or
philosophical inquiry; and in which even the
good and the true are pursued with an ardor
more indicative of nervous excitement than of
pure, unadulterated emotion. The prevalent feeling is, that whatever is worth striving for at all,
is worthy of all possible zeal and devotion ; and,
supported by the sympathy and coöperation of
others similarly disposed, the coldest natures be-

come, at last, willing to go as far and as fast as
any. Indeed, a man can hardly gain the credit
of honesty in his opinions, unless ever ready to
surrender himself soul and body to their support.
Where the mind of a person revolves in a very
narrow circle of thought, it lacks entirely that
recuperative and invigorating power which
springs from a wider comprehension of things,
and more numerous objects of interest. The
habit of brooding over a single idea is calculated
to dwarf the soundest mind; but to those unfortunately constituted, it is positively dangerous,
because they are easily led to this kind of partial mental activity, and are kept from running
into fatal extremes by none of those conservative
agencies which a broader discipline and a more
generous culture naturally furnish. The result
of this continual dwelling on a favorite idea is,
that it comes up unbidden, and cannot be dismissed at pleasure. Reason, fancy, passion,
emotion, — every power of the mind, in short, —
are pressed into its service, until it is magnified
into gigantic proportions and endowed with
wonderful attributes. The conceptions become
unnaturally vivid, the general views narrow and
distorted, the proprieties of time and place are
disregarded, the guiding, controlling power of
the mind is disturbed, and, as the last stage of
this melancholy process, reason is completely

dethroned. These persons should be careful, therefore, how they suffer themselves to be led into the active support of those prominent moral and social enterprises that abound in every community. No matter what may be their convictions touching the necessity or justice of these projects, or the claims they make on the sympathy of all good and true men. They cannot join the ranks of those whose devotion to their favorite cause knows no stint or measure, without serious peril to their mental integrity. Let them, therefore, habitually feel that their mission in life lies in the quiet, unobtrusive performance of those duties which are incumbent on all, rather than in the promotion of enterprises which court the public gaze and stimulate their energies to the highest possible pitch. Let them not be beguiled by any fanciful obligations of duty, to quit the humbler sphere of effort most suitable to their mental capacities. There will always be enough to take the prominent places which they had better avoid, while no sphere of life is without its opportunities of useful and honorable effort.

Man is a creature, not only of intellect and appetite, but of sentiment. He is endowed with faculties whereby certain attributes of men and things excite emotions of pleasure or pain, — all necessary to the accomplishment of the

ends of his existence, — all essential to his happiness as a moral and rational creature, — all
essential to the maintenance of his responsibility to God and man. That the sentiments, as
well as the intellect, may be perverted by disease, is a fact to which the phenomena of insanity abundantly testify. There is no reason why
they should not. Indeed, since the intellectual
and moral faculties are equally dependent on
the brain, the manifestations of cerebral disorder
are as likely to appear in one as in the other.
Which it may happen to be, is a question, I apprehend, of cerebral locality, and, it may be, of
certain organic conditions not yet understood.
It is not disputed that disease may affect the
intellect, without, at the same time, involving,
apparently, the affective powers; and it is no
less obvious that the latter may be greatly disordered while the former *seems*, at least, to remain in its normal condition. To say that
mental disease necessarily implies obvious intellectual aberration, is simply to ignore the
testimony of every day's observation. The
question is not, whether, in such cases, the intellect is entirely untouched by the disease, but
whether or not the disease is so slight as to
escape notice, and thus not sensibly affect the
great predominance of the moral disorder. If
we were contending against a barren specula-

20

tion, it would be labor lost, no doubt; but the practical consequences of the doctrine cannot be regarded without the deepest concern. So long as the intellect is not visibly diseased, it is alleged, there is no insanity, — none certainly that can impair the legal responsibility of the patient. Disease may sap the very foundations of the moral nature; it may blast the sentiments of benevolence, of justice, of veneration,—changing naturally mild and amiable dispositions into malignant passions; converting the man of generous, open-hearted nature, into a miser, with no thought of anything but accumulation; the man of sternest integrity into a pilferer of the smallest description; the staid, quiet, respectable citizen into a noisy, shameless brawler, regardless of every rule of common propriety or courtesy, — and yet, in no court of conscience or of justice, is he to claim any exemption from the ordinary consequences of vice and crime! Surely, it is a monstrous doctrine to put forth in an age of humanity and science, that just when those moral checks and balances which the Creator has placed in the human soul, for the proper ordering of the life and the attainment of life's great ends, are disarranged and perverted by the intrusion of a foreign element, the individual is none the less capable of performing his moral duties and obligations, and none the less accountable for any short-comings that may follow. It is difficult to argue against a doctrine so destitute of any foundation in fact, and opposed to the testimony of every day's observation; and one is obliged to be contented with simply an expression of wonder and amazement.

If, indeed, the moral powers hold such intimate relations with mental disease, then, certainly, the discipline to which they are subjected becomes a matter of the highest importance. Bearing in mind the fundamental law of the animal economy, that excessive exercise of a faculty leads to its disease, all the more surely and speedily when the conservative power is weakened by hereditary tendency to disease, we may readily understand the necessity of prudence in the use of those faculties, on the part of persons thus constituted. In some degree, at least, they have the power of controlling their moral movements, and, to that extent, of hastening or retarding an attack of disease; and some, — a small proportion, perhaps, but large enough to be worth saving, if possible, — need only to be put on their guard in order to avoid the danger.

To know where their danger lies, let them ascertain, not only by self-examination, but by the counsel of judicious friends, their own ruling sentiments, — those which determine, in a great degree, their peculiar traits of character. No one sees himself exactly as others see him, and none hit so wide of a proper self-estimate, as those whose insight is disturbed by the play of morbid tendencies. Let the persons in question distrust themselves, therefore, and defer to the judgment of others who are competent to observe correctly their mental peculiarities, and are moved by a sincere interest in their welfare. Thus may they learn the impending danger in season to avoid it, and before the world at large, perhaps, is aware of its existence.

When mental disease is fairly established, it becomes a matter of professional care, but before it is fully developed, and in some degree afterwards, much must be left, in regard to its moral and domestic management, to the intelligence and discretion of friends. To perform their duty properly, in a position of so much responsibility, and under such unusual relations, they need especial advice and direction. On the course they pursue may depend the fate of a wife, a child, a parent, a friend; and therefore they should be governed by reliable information rather than by vulgar prejudice and ignorance. In the progress of the disease, from the first barely perceptible wandering to unequivocal disorder, there comes a time when those nearest and dearest to the patient are bound by every consideration of propriety and humanity to assume some control over his actions. The exact moment when this step should be taken, in any given case, is not easily settled, and thus the mistake is not unfrequently made, either of interfering too soon, and thus precipitating the evil we are seeking to avert, or, as is far more common, waiting until some sad occurrence takes place, or the favorable season for arresting the course of the malady is irretrievably lost. General directions on this subject must be too indefinite to admit of very exact practical application, but they will serve, at the least, to indicate the duty in question, and the importance of performing it rightly.

The early stage of insanity, or its *incubation*, as it is professionally called,—that which precedes a degree of mental impairment that disqualifies the person from maintaining his ordinary relations to others, — may be long or short, embracing a period of years, or only of a few days or weeks. It may consist in a few oddities of behavior or changes of affection, of little practical moment, or in irregular conduct, or unaccountable dislikes, or simple idleness and loss of all power of application to business, or a disposition to embark in all manner of schemes and enterprises; in an apathy that no persuasion can shake, or a restlessness manifested in incessant roaming; in excessive hilarity that surprises rather than grieves, or a deep despondency that leads to self-destruction. No single rule of management can be applicable to such a variety of conditions, but a few hints may be of some practical service.

Indications of intended violence, especially towards those whose relations to the patient place them completely within his power, will justify immediate interference, however correct and rational otherwise he may appear. To wait until some overt act of violence is committed, is no kindness to him, but gross injustice. Most of those terrible acts which excite a thrill of horror through whole communities, are committed by this very class of the insane, whose unsoundness does not seem, to timid, hesitating friends, sufficient to warrant any measure of restraint.

Again, when mental disorder consists in a kind of exaltation manifested in loud and extravagant discourse, not proper for the public ear; or in a disposition to ramble about without regard to the ordinary proprieties of place and season; or in a fondness for bargains or commercial enterprises unsuited to the natural habits, tastes, or means, then interference is needed to save the patient from jeopardizing

health, reputation, or fortune, and exposing his
infirmity in a manner calculated to cause him,
when he comes to himself, unspeakable grief and
mortification. In the opposite condition, too,
where the mind is overwhelmed by distressing
doubts and apprehensions, joined perhaps to a
sense of utter unworthiness, with not a single
ray of hope in the future, the shortest delay is
dangerous, because the patient invariably thinks
of self-destruction as a means of relief. It may
be only a thought never ripening into execution,
or an impulse steadily gathering force until it
becomes irresistible. Many a case of suicide
which bursts upon the public notice like thunder from a cloudless sky, is the result of this
inexcusable reluctance on the part of friends, to
impose restraint on one who seems to be suffering merely a fit of low spirits.

These, by way of example, are a few of the
mental conditions which justify and even demand interference, before the person betrays unequivocal proof of insanity. In respect to that
large class of cases the circumstances of which
furnish room for reasonable doubt, but little
more can be said beyond enjoining upon those
on whom the responsibility rests, unceasing vigilance and circumspection, and assuring them
that, although premature interference may be
an evil, yet a far greater may result from mis-
placed delay.

The object proposed by interference is to place the party under suitable restraint, and subject him to the requisite moral and medical treatment. In selecting the particular form of the measure, reference must always be had to the circumstances of the case — to the grade of the disorder, the disposition of the patient, his domestic relations, and pecuniary condition. The nature of the malady is incompatible with that ready acquiescence in the wishes of friends which is generally yielded in other disorders; and, therefore, those wishes must be enforced by means more peremptory than arguments. Such means may be used, occasionally, in the patient's own home, in the midst of his family, and occasionally they may prove sufficient for the purpose. He yields to the measures thought necessary for his safety and restoration, makes no attempt to escape from control, and is harmless to himself and others. But, for the most part, domestic supervision is not thorough enough to obviate all danger from the disordered passions, and sentiments; or the patient rebels against the mildest form of restraint; or he is too obstinate or too apathetic to follow the prescribed treatment. In such cases, it becomes necessary to choose some form of restraint more stringent and effectual. This is sometimes obtained by placing him in some other family than his own, in the hope that he will yield to strangers or less familiar acquaintances what he refuses to his immediate friends. Occasionally, the result is favorable. The withdrawal from painful associations, and the presence of those whose favor and authority are not to be slighted, render him sufficiently docile, and the new position exerts a decidedly salutary influence. Generally, however, this measure proves as ineffectual as the management at home, and is liable to the same objections.

In the early stage of the disease travelling is often recommended, especially by medical men, who suppose that the necessary presence of a companion furnishes all the required restraint, and that the impressions produced by frequent change of scene may exert a restorative influence. The reasons offered for this course are so plausible, and the authority by which it is recommended so imposing, that, where the means are not wanting, it is oftener resorted to than any other. I will not say that it is never successful, for that would be hardly correct; but such a result, according to my observation, is exceedingly rare, and a little reflection on the mental condition will show us the reason. The truth is that, whether excited or depressed, the mind is strongly exercised by the strange thoughts and emotions that possess it. It needs rest, repose, withdrawal from excitement, or at most, a kind of

activity which is carefully measured and directed
by an experienced head. It is not in a condition
to be gratified by external impressions, while
their frequency and variety rather disturb and
distract the thoughts, than turn them into healthier channels. By that kind of vicious association which characterizes the operations of the
insane mind, these impressions only serve to give
additional force and vividness to its unnatural
conceptions. In every new face, perhaps, it
sees a confirmation of its suspicions; in every
untoward incident, new food for its painful apprehensions; in every arrangement, some special
reference to its own condition. In the few cases
where travelling has been beneficial, I am inclined to think that the disorder was in its very
earliest stage, consisting in an inability to govern the thoughts at all times, or only a little
dejection of spirits or disinclination to mental
effort. Probably, it would oftener succeed were
it tried thus early, instead of being deferred, as
it usually is, until the disease is firmly fixed.

The very natural reluctance to take a step
which unequivocally recognizes the actual presence of insanity, induces the friends to resort to
other measures, even more inappropriate, if not
more mischievous, than travelling. In the belief
or hope which they fondly cherish, that the
disorder is only a form of hysteria, or a little

temporary disturbance of mind resulting from a cold or a menstrual suppression, which will shortly disappear, they send the patient to some noted spring, water-cure, or other establishment that promises health and longevity to every suffering child of Adam. I fear that medical men too often encourage this flattering unction, and lend the sanction of their authority to measures of which the mildest censure that can be uttered is that they are generally fruitless. It is an ungrateful, it is a painful office, to dissipate the last delusive hope, and announce a dread reality; but here the highest interest of the patient and the friends implicitly require the plain, unvarnished truth.

There remains to be considered one more instrumentality for guarding and restoring the disordered mind, viz: establishments designed expressly for the custody and cure of the insane — an end which they have fulfilled with a degree of success which has rendered them prominent among the triumphs of modern philanthropy and science. Their object is to provide the necessary restraint in a manner as little disagreeable as possible, and furnish the necessary treatment at a price within the means of the humblest classes, and with a kind of skill that can be obtained only from special observation and training. By many, however, they are regarded with

distrust and aversion, for they cannot see what
there is in a hospital, even when faithfully managed, capable of compensating for the absence
of those attentions and conveniences which are
supposed to be found only in one's own home.
To sever a man's domestic ties, to take him out
of the circle of friends and relatives most deeply
interested in his welfare and ready to spend and
be spent for his sake, at the very moment too
when his mind is distracted with jealousy and
suspicion, and bodily infirmity perhaps has rendered him more or less helpless, and place him
beyond the reach of a very close observation, in
the hands of strangers, and in the company of
persons as disordered as himself — all this, at
first sight, would seem as little likely to exert a
restorative effect as any course that could possibly be devised.   Right views on this subject are
so important, that I shall be but serving the
purpose in hand, to explain with some particularity the peculiar advantages of hospitals for
the insane over other means for treating this
disease.

Insanity implies the existence of bodily derangement, and therefore is a suitable object of
medical treatment, which, of course, would be
more skilfully applied by men who are devoting their whole time and attention to this affection, than by those who observe it only on a

very limited scale. But it also implies derangement of the ideas, hallucination of the senses,
perversion of the moral sentiments, all which,
though the result of physical disorder, are, so
far as their outward manifestations are concerned, in some degree, under the control of
others, and by such control — in a way not very
well understood — the morbid process may be
arrested. Now, it is the moral management
prevalent in the hospitals of our own time,
which so strongly distinguishes them from
those of any former time, and determines, in a
great measure, the amount of good which they
accomplish. Until within a comparatively recent period, insanity was treated by medical
men very much like other diseases. Regarding
it only in its physical aspect, they considered
their duty as finished when they had exhausted
the kind of medication supposed to be most
efficacious for the purpose. But in an age
of active philanthropy and of great practical
sagacity, the idea was not long in making its
appearance, that something more is necessary to
insure the highest success, even to the medical
treatment. The fact was finally recognized that
so long as the patient is allowed to follow the
bent of his own will, he is only fostering and
strengthening the morbid process going on in
the brain ; and it also became obvious that or-

dinary nurses in private families or in general
hospitals are incompetent to exercise the kind
of control which the case required. Seldom
seeing the disease, they have little opportunity
of acquiring skill in the practice of their duty;
and, besides, even if it were otherwise, it could
not be expected that persons of their capacity
and culture could ever do more than follow,
with more or less fidelity, the general directions of others. These directions the medical
attendant could not furnish, because he knew
comparatively little of the disease himself, and
had given no special attention to the operations
of the mind whether sane or insane. Visiting
his patient at infrequent intervals, he could not
provide for his frequently changing moods, nor
be sure that his views were faithfully executed.
Neither would the arrangements of an ordinary
household admit of that kind of restriction
which the insane usually require, and the only
alternative was, either an unlimited indulgence
of the patient in his caprices, or a degree of
coercion and confinement which irritated his
spirit and injured his health. Under the pressure of these inconveniences and hindrances, the
idea began to prevail that the insane could be
best managed in establishments devoted exclusively to their care. It was obvious that persons engaged in their service would become

familiar with the ways of the insane, and thereby learn a thousand arts of management, and
acquire a degree of skill in the performance of
their duties, quite unknown to others. The
medical man, too, concentrating his attention
upon a single disease, and devoting all his time
to the little community around him, would obtain an amount of practical information which
no other source can supply. He would also
impart to the general management of an establishment a kind of efficiency which can only
spring from continuous and systematic effort
conducted upon a large scale. The latter result was rendered probable by the example of
general hospitals, where congregations of similar cases afford unusual means for studying
their nature and obtaining the highest possible
degree of skill in their treatment. The world
has not been disappointed. The beneficial results expected from special hospitals for the
insane have been abundantly experienced, and
the benevolence of the age has been largely
engaged in establishing them, until they have
become firmly rooted in the necessities and
affections of every Christian community.

We have already intimated that their superior success in the treatment of the insane
depends, chiefly, on the greater efficiency of
their moral management. It is one of their

merits, indeed, that this management works so
easily, and substitutes so quietly its own arrangements for the suggestions of disease, that
the uninitiated observer finds it difficult to appreciate its real value, and thus often mistakes
the character of its results. He sees the patient
taking no medicine, perhaps; calm in his discourse and movements; readily complying with
the wishes of others; and engaging, it may be,
in some form of work or amusement; and he
adopts the conclusion, which no opinion of the
physician can shake, that the patient has recovered, or, at any rate, is so much better, that he
would do equally well at home or in a private
family. He can scarcely be made to believe
that what he witnesses is chiefly the result of
that special management peculiar to a modern
hospital for the insane; of architectural arrangements which restrain without annoyance;
of systematic regularity in the daily routine of
life; of gentle manners; judicious firmness; vigilant, enlightened, and conscientious supervision.
Now, these qualities are not a matter of accident, nor are they the growth of a day. They
are the elaborated result of a profound study
of the mental constitution both in health and
disease; of extensive inquiry into the various
arts concerned in the erection and practical
working of a considerable establishment; and

of an organization of the service best calculated to effect its destined object. To suppose them otherwise would be to commit a folly like that of inferring from the quiet, easy working of a complicated machine, that its construction is very simple and was readily accomplished; thus overlooking entirely the years of meditation, the numberless experiments, and the successive steps towards the desired object, that finally led to an admirable piece of mechanism.

The peculiar restlessness of the insane which impels them to roam about regardless of time and occasion, at the risk of their own safety and the peace of society, and which finds no sufficient restriction in the arrangements of an ordinary dwelling short of confinement in a small apartment, is effectually controlled in a hospital; while the range of ample galleries and airing-courts prevents that control from being oppressive and unhealthy. Their fitful humors, their wild caprices, their impulsive movements, their angry looks, are met by the steady and straightforward will of attendants who have learned to perform their duty unbiased by fear or favor. Having no object of their own to serve; imbibing the spirit of kindness which prevails around them; deterred from improper practices by a vigilant supervision, and aided by suitable architectural con-

21

trivances, they are enabled to manage their charge with the least possible degree of annoyance. Thus withdrawn from outward excitements, and especially from the persons and scenes connected with his mental disorder, the patient naturally becomes calmer, his mind opens to better suggestions, and finally seeks for repose in amusement or labor. And thus it happens that in many cases but little more is necessary to conduct the morbid process to a successful issue, besides giving the constitution a fair chance to exert its restorative powers, unembarrassed by adverse influences.

In the hospital, the patient is withdrawn from the countless adverse incidents to which he is elsewhere exposed. He is saved from the advice of good-natured friends, oftener pernicious than salutary, because founded on very imperfect notions of insanity; he is saved from hearing or seeing something every hour calculated to maintain the morbid process which is nourished by what might seem to be the most harmless material; he is saved from all those disagreeable associations between the morbid thoughts and emotions, and the scenes, persons, and objects around him, which serve, in the strongest manner, to perpetuate the mental disturbance. The importance of the last consideration is not generally understood; many, no doubt, are not even aware of its existence. It is now a well-settled principle, that, to treat the insane with the highest degree of success, the surroundings of the patient should be entirely changed, so that he shall see no face nor other object familiar to him in the previous stage of his disease, nor recognize anything in fact calculated to remind him by force of association, of some distressing thought or feeling. For we must bear in mind that even in cases where we should least expect it, the sight of some trivial object, — a door, a paper-hanging, or a piece of furniture, or the hearing of some unmeaning sound, — is suggesting, it may be, a train of uncomfortable reflections. They who have charge of hospitals for the insane will tell us that the sight of a bundle of old clothes from home is sufficient to reproduce all the original excitement and agitation in many a patient, calm, quiet, and apparently convalescing. In these things, we find the explanation of the common fact of the immediate and considerable improvement following the removal of the patient from his own home to the hospital.

The domestic management of the insane is most at fault in failing to meet the successive changes in their condition with appropriate treatment, and especially in permitting a premature withdrawal from seclusion. The earli-

est symptom of returning reason is the signal
for removing restrictions, and the first intima-
tion from the patient of a wish to visit his
customary haunts and engage in his customary
pursuits is cheerfully gratified; and even if the
friends should suspect the propriety of the
course, their better judgment is overborne by
the importunity of the patient. But his brain
is still irritable, and easily disturbed by new and
various emotions. A short experience shows that
the trial is beyond his powers; the morbid process is reproduced, and soon assumes its original severity, and he is fortunate indeed if he
ever recover the ground he has lost. That
this is a frequent result of domestic management we have abundant reason to believe, and
no degree of intelligence or discretion on the
part of friends could well make it otherwise.
In the hospital, on the contrary, this stage of
the disease, when the cloud is beginning to
disperse, is as carefully watched as any other,
and the skill of the physician is no less required to conduct it to unequivocal convales-
cence. The patient's incessant solicitations for
release are met by a firm denial; his impatience and discontent, however urgently manifested, are unable to prevail against a strong
sense of duty and a clear apprehension of his
true condition. Even in the limited intercourse

which the patient while in the hospital maintains with his friends, he often succeeds in
bending them to his wishes. It is precisely
in this transition period of the disease, when
its graver effects have been succeeded by a
morbid irritability of the brain, producing unusual restlessness and impatience, — the period
when, of all others, is needed their willing co-
operation, because the patient's hopes and efforts to obtain his release are then the greatest
obstacles to be encountered in the work of restoration, — it is just then, I say, that one has
the most occasion to deplore their misjudged
interference. He admits that he was very ill
when he came in, but declares that he has recovered entirely, and was never better in his
life; for he eats, works, and feels, as well as ever,
and that it is downright cruelty and oppression
to keep him from his family and business. He
appeals to their affection and their sense of
right, and, to quicken their sympathies in his
behalf, he may insinuate that his treatment in
the hospital is not exactly what they would
approve. In the severer grades of this condition, he may even endeavor to excite their apprehensions by the fearful prediction that he
will soon become a fool or a maniac like the
rest of them. Too often, friends are moved by
such appeals from those they love and respect.

They try to persuade themselves that such discontent is worse than any possible consequences of a premature removal; they fear to incur the patient's displeasure; and finally work themselves into the belief that the doctor is unnecessarily scrupulous — perhaps governed by interested views. Now, we know that this trait which makes so strong an impression on them is one of the most common phenomena of insanity, and is indicative of *morbid action in the brain.* We also know that under a longer perseverance it will finally disappear, and be succeeded by a calm and contented spirit in which the patient has less confidence in his own strength, and is more willing to be guided by the advice of others. We also know that a return to customary scenes and pursuits will only aggravate rather than relieve this restless feeling, and in a large proportion of cases, he goes back in a condition less promising than the first. I have no hesitation in saying that many of the incurables that form so large a share of the inmates of our hospitals, have been made so by the interference of well-meaning but injudicious friends.

It is well understood, except, of course, by those who are governed by the most vulgar prejudices, that the moral management in hospitals for the insane is characterized by invari

able mildness, unmingled with any of that severity which was once regarded as indispensable,
yet but few understand precisely how it is
maintained. It would seem, from the common
notion on this subject, that, the correctness of
the principle once recognized,• nothing more
would be necessary to insure a practical ful-
filment. Men make no account of any possible conflict between principle and practice,
and forget the influence of deficient culture
and the force of passion. They do not seem
to be aware that, under the circumstances of
the case, the supremacy of the moral sentiments can be maintained only by special management, and that if the discipline of a hospital
is very different from that of a jail or a poor-
house, the fact cannot be attributed to chance.
If this point were well understood, hospitals
would be more correctly appreciated than they
can be under merely general impressions of
their utility, and therefore it may be worth our
while to advert to it for a moment.

The rules of these institutions enjoin upon all
engaged in the service, the uniform observance
of a mild and gentle deportment, and forbid
the use of harsh words and rough handling,
under pain of dismissal. This is one step towards the object, but, without something more,
it would scarcely be sufficient to gain it. To

make the rule an active, vital principle, pervading every part of the service upon the patients,
infusing itself into the morals and manners of
all, prompting every movement and character-
izing every effort, softening the tones and looks,
and inspiring confidence and self-respect, — to
save it, in short, from becoming a mere dead
letter, — the service must be organized and directed in a benevolent and elevated spirit, by
men who are led by their own discipline and
culture to enforce a rigid performance of duty,
and possess the requisite qualities of mind for
carrying their views into practical effect. In
this way, and in this only, will the service be
pervaded by a high moral feeling, if that may
be called so which is the result of a system
rather than a spontaneous or conscientious effort. In considerable establishments, the high
character of the service is the result of special
training and careful supervision. The attendant, on entering upon his duty, readily falls into
the established routine, and yields to the influences around him. He is directed by others
who know more than himself, and his own discretion and temper are exercised within very
narrow limits. By precept and example, he
learns that he is engaged in an honorable service, and is naturally led to magnify his office.
From this feeling there arises an *esprit du corps*,

a sort of public sentiment, which elevates his aims, and rebukes improper practices more effectually than a code of regulations. In the private family, on the contrary, all is very different. There the attendant is virtually supreme, for the power above him may know no better than he what the exigencies of the case require, and hence his charge is exposed to injurious indulgences or unnecessary restrictions. Unwatched, and unimpressed by surrounding influences, there is nothing to prevent him from yielding to his impulses under irritation, and venting his spleen upon the patient. If recovery takes place under such circumstances, it must be in spite of attendance, and not at all in consequence of any restorative influence exerted by it.

If it be asked wherein this peculiar character of hospital service is manifested, I would point to a few particular instances. It is evinced in a regard for cleanliness and proprieties of dress, which is so necessary in maintaining the self-respect of the patient, and which is preserved only by dint of unceasing attention. When the mind is deeply involved in disease, this is almost the first of the minor virtues to disappear, and its loss prepares the way for others of a more serious character. In the common observances of life, in the incoming and the outgoing,

in the uprising and the downlying, in partaking
of meals, engaging in exercise or amusement,
the effect of the attendance is visible in the regularity and quiet and good order with which
those things are managed. In many cases this
alone, apparently, is sufficient to calm the turbu-
lence of the excited, and produce some attempt
at self-control. In another instance, it is witnessed in the facility with which the patients
are controlled, as is shown in the remarkably
little amount of mechanical restraint which is
used. Once the management of the insane
was inseparable from the idea of handcuffs,
strait-jackets, and strong-chairs. It is scarcely
twenty years since chains were abolished in the
hospitals of London; and in private practice,
some form of restraint was rather the rule than
the exception. It was supposed that such
means were necessary to insure the safety of
all concerned, but it is now well understood
that, by vigilance and tact, they may be almost
entirely dispensed with, while just so much will
be gained in maintaining the good nature and
self-respect of the patient. In short, the great
ends of moral treatment, — quiet, self-control,
orderly and respectful behavior, confidence in
others, submission to a higher will, — may all
be witnessed in well-regulated hospitals for the
insane, as the result of a moral management

characterized by judicious firmness and invariable kindness.

Our duties to the patient do not end when he is placed in a hospital. Even there, though not under our immediate care, he is still, or ought to be, the object of our unceasing, but judicious supervision; and upon the manner in which this duty is performed depends, in some degree, the result of the measure.

In the first place, it should be allowed to have a fair trial. Comparatively few are aware that insanity is very variable, and, at best, not very short in its duration. People are apt to imagine that it runs its course as rapidly as a fever; or, at any rate, that the magical influences of a hospital will cut it short. They expect that amendment will soon follow, and become impatient if it is long delayed. The fact is, that weeks, months, and oftentimes years, may elapse, without recovery or even improvement. Statistics show that a large portion of the recoveries occur in the second or third year after the attack. The delay of improvement, therefore, even for a considerable period, is an insufficient reason for impatience or loss of confidence. Let the friends beware how they adopt the conclusion that the experiment has failed, and that they are bound to try some other. I unhesitatingly say, on the strength of

much observation, that in many a person the
disease has been made permanent in consequence of precipitate removal, who would probably have recovered under a persevering trial of
hospital treatment. I do not mean to convey
the idea that any man's judgment is infallible or
to be implicitly followed, but rather that change
of management should be always prompted,
not by whim, nor caprice, nor the suggestions of that large class of worthies who, with
a degree of confidence equalled only by that
of their ignorance, are always ready to volunteer
advice in the affairs of their neighbors, but by
reasons founded on exact knowledge of the
nature of the disease as affected by outward
influences and associations.

Another duty incumbent on the friends is, to
refrain from all interference with the medical or
moral management of the patient. This should
be entrusted without reserve to the physician,
and a thorough compliance with his wishes will
best promote the desired object. Many a person who would never think of questioning the
correctness of the medical treatment, will insist
on following his own judgment rather than the
physician's, in respect to that most important
part of all moral management, the intercourse
of the patient with his friends. And yet, in the
process of restoration, it is well understood that

drugs, valuable as they are in their place, are far less efficacious than those incidents and influences that act directly on the brain. It is hard to believe, no doubt, that those who are nearly related to the sufferer should refrain from visiting him when he seems to be in most need of comfort and consolation; but a little reflection on the subject will show, that what would be a sacred duty under ordinary circumstances, may be a source of serious mischief here.

Let it be considered that the principal advantage possessed by a hospital over every other means of treating the insane is, that it secures most perfectly their seclusion from whatever tends to produce excessive emotion. While at large, the patient is every moment exposed to circumstances that maintain the morbid activity of his mind and strengthen his aberrations; and in his diseased condition, almost everything in which his feelings are deeply interested has this effect. In the hospital, on the contrary, he is beyond the reach of all these causes of excitement, and thus nature is allowed to exert its healing influences without any hindrance from without. Quiet, silence, regular routine, take the place of restlessness, noise, and fitful activity; and, instead of receiving a variety of impressions calculated to excite and distract, he moves in a certain monotonous round, which, however dis-

agreeable to sane men, may be absolutely necessary to the restoration of a disordered mind.
To a person laboring under any degree of maniacal excitement, and to many of those also
whose aberrations are of a depressing character,
the sight of old friends, especially after a long
separation, stimulates the mental movements
already beyond control. By calling up a host
of old associations, by exciting painful, or even
pleasurable suggestions, the vital movements of
the brain are precipitated, the excitement which
had been allayed by the temporary seclusion is
kindled afresh, and thus the hold of disease is
strengthened. The dearer the friend, the greater
the emotion. The same person who would
meet a stranger with comparative indifference,
might be agitated beyond control by the sight
and conversation of those who are bound to
them by ties of blood and affection. It is a
great mistake to suppose that the insane are in-
juriously affected only by such as they dislike,
and that the visits of those to whom they are
tenderly attached cannot be otherwise than
soothing and salutary. It is not so much the
character as the strength of the emotion, which
does the injury; and, therefore, even the pleasing as well as the painful emotions may, by
means of the associations connected with them,
prove too much for the disordered reason. So

susceptible is the patient rendered by the extreme irritability which is a common feature of insanity, that, as already observed, the receipt of a parcel from home, especially if it be some familiar object, often produces agitation and disturbance not readily allayed.

Another duty of friends is, not to precipitate the discharge of the patient merely because all trace of disease seems to have vanished. After the more demonstrative signs of insanity have disappeared, a certain grade of disease may still exist, though not obvious on a casual inspection. The patient receives his friends courteously, eagerly inquires for others, expresses an interest in persons and things at home, declares he was never better in his life, and his whole air and manner seem to confirm the assertion. By the partial judgment of friends, the object of seclusion is regarded as fully accomplished, and no reason is supposed to exist for separating him any longer from family and home. They, however, who see him from day to day, watch his ways, and listen to his discourse, know very well that traces of delusion still linger in his mind; that the current of his affections is far from smooth and clear, and that he imperfectly appreciates both his past and present condition. And experience tells them that only a longer probation is required to complete the restoration which removal would be likely to prevent altogether. Under these circumstances, friends are much inclined to think that the physician is unduly cautious, and that farther seclusion would only disquiet and irritate, rather than exert a restorative influence. Accordingly, the impatience and importunity of the patient are allowed too frequently to prevail over the counsels of the physician, and the step is taken which, oftener than otherwise, results in disappointment and sorrow. The sudden change from a state of complete subjection to the control of others to that of complete self-dependence, requires a degree of vigor and elasticity which the brain does not possess. The sight of familiar scenes and objects and faces revives a host of painful associations not very conducive to recovery, and even strengthens and fixes delusions that were steadily passing away. The self-confidence which usually characterizes this condition, brooks no check nor caution from those who have no power to enforce their wishes, and leads to efforts and enterprises quite beyond reach. One indiscretion is followed by another; the conservative principles of the brain, one after another, are lost; until, at last, in full view of anxious friends, powerless to prevent or delay the result, the empire of disease becomes fully reëstablished.

It should be borne in mind that, in most cases, the restorative process, from the first signs of improvement to complete, genuine recovery, occupies a considerable period, and is marked by many fluctuations. In this disease, the vital movements are governed by a law of periodicity, more or less regular, in consequence of which, time is generally required, in order to determine exactly the character of any change, whether for better or worse. The most decided improvement may prove to be only a remission in the severity of the disease; only one in a cycle of changes in which the morbid movement may revolve. And at the best, the brain is long in regaining its normal hardihood, and until it does, exemption from relapse, under any circumstances of trial, cannot be confidently expected. A person who, after spraining his ankle, should undertake to walk a mile or two the moment all pain and inflammation had disappeared, would be regarded as committing a great folly. To use one's brain immediately after the demonstrative symptoms of insanity have passed away, as if all its powers were completely restored, is a folly so much the greater as the brain is so much the more delicate and susceptible than the tendons and cartilages of the ankle. When precisely a patient can, with safety, be restored to his family and customary pursuits, is a ques-

22

tion which, beyond all others in the treatment of
the insane, will task the resources of the professional man to answer correctly. It is the part
of wisdom, then, to leave it always to him, with
the consoling reflection, that if, in prolonging
the probation, he errs, it is, unquestionably, an
error on the safe side. Many recovered persons
say they left the hospital too soon — that they
were far from being well when they left —
though apparently restored to their normal condition, while the few who complain of having
been kept too long, were obviously removed before they were restored.